THE **COMPLETE GUIDE** TO
MASSAGE

A STEP-BY-STEP GUIDE to achieving the health and relaxation benefits of massage

Edited by **Mary Biancalana**, MS, CMTPT, LMT, CPT

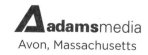
Aadamsmedia
Avon, Massachusetts

Published by
Adams Media, a division of F+W Media, Inc.
57 Littlefield Street, Avon, MA 02322. U.S.A.
www.adamsmedia.com

Contains material adapted from *The Everything® Massage Book* by Valerie Voner, LMT, CRT, RMT,
copyright © 2004 by F+W Media, Inc., ISBN 10: 1-59337-071-7, ISBN 13: 978-1-59337-071-8.

ISBN 10: 1-4405-9401-5
ISBN 13: 978-1-4405-9401-4
eISBN 10: 1-4405-9402-3
eISBN 13: 978-1-4405-9402-1

Printed in the United States of America.

10 9 8 7 6 5 4 3 2 1

The Complete Guide to Massage is intended as a reference volume only, not as a medical or fitness manual. The ideas, procedures, and suggestions in this book are intended to supplement, not replace, the advice of a trained medical professional. Consult your physician about any condition that may require medical attention before adopting the suggestions and programs in this book. The author and publisher disclaim any liability arising directly or indirectly from the use of this book.

Many of the designations used by manufacturers and sellers to distinguish their products are claimed as trademarks. Where those designations appear in this book and F+W Media, Inc. was aware of a trademark claim, the designations have been printed with initial capital letters.

Cover design by Sylvia McArdle.
Cover photographs by iStockphoto.com/MarsBars and Deana Travers, Home Town Photo.
Interior photographs by Deana Travers, Home Town Photo.

This book is available at quantity discounts for bulk purchases.
For information, please call 1-800-289-0963.

Contents

Introduction

From the dawn of humankind, humans have recognized the importance and comfort of touch. Massage is the natural inclination to touch, to soothe, to rub, or to take away or ease whatever ails you. Massage is also a form of communication; you can use it to actually talk to someone without words. When you are gently rubbing the tired arms and hands of a beloved partner, you are expressing your feelings through the compassion of your touch. This book will show you how to use massage on yourself and to share its gifts with others.

Touch through massage is a way to share yourself with others. A relationship of honor and trust is established through the give-and-take of caring touch. To receive massage is to trust the giver, and to give massage is to honor the receiver. The knowledge you gain from this book will contribute to improving your relationship with yourself as well as with others. You are opening a door to whole wellness as you study educated touch, visualizing your hands as tools of healing. Massage takes away aches and pains while providing comfort in the most basic of our instincts, touch.

Massage is used today in a variety of settings. Everyone from athletes to infants to businesspeople can benefit from massage. Massage is used in physical therapy and in specific treatment of certain medical conditions. Massage has become popular in many areas of healing, including nursing care and spa treatments. It is used by doctors to alleviate problems in the least invasive way, and without drugs.

We discuss in this book the different strokes and movements within a massage, and explore the variety of massages available, giving you an array of choices. As you develop an informed touch, your fingers will know what to do on the body you are massaging.

Massage can be as fancy or as simple as you make it. Giving a massage is pleasurable and can be done anywhere; it takes only two people—a giver and a receiver. Whether you are outside or indoors, at home or at work, have a free afternoon or a quick lunch break, performing and receiving massage is nearly always a possibility.

Through the study and examination of massage, you find that the physical and emotional relaxation you experience as a receiver and a giver frees your spirit. Welcome to the world of joyous giving.

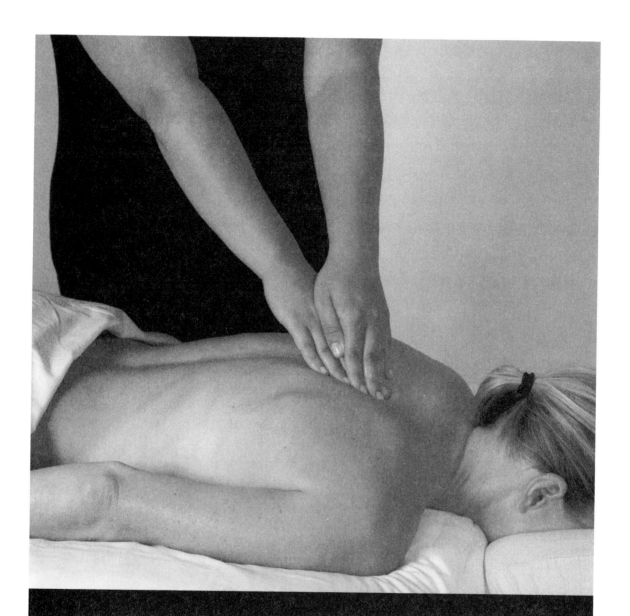

Part 1 **The Fundamentals**

Chapter 1

What Is Massage?

Understanding What Massage Is

Massage is the manipulation of soft tissue and muscle in the support of natural healing, using hands, arms, and fingers as the tools. Anyone thinking about massage usually conjures up a mental picture of one person relaxing and another person applying smooth, steady strokes to promote further relaxation. The skin is the perfect palette for massage. In fact, your intuitive response to pain, whether physical or emotional, is to rub the offending area in an effort to soothe away the pain. Massage is simply an organized expression of your own natural instinct and ability.

Massage promotes holistic health, which is the balance of body, mind, and spirit in a healthy, drug-free environment. This systematic application of healing touch creates an environment of balance that in turn fosters good health. Massage may provide relaxation or stimulation, depending upon the techniques used. Massage encourages joy and happiness, for both the receiver and the giver. In short, massage is a key to enhancing your well-being.

> **Massage for Self-Healing**
>
> Our bodies have an innate gift—the capacity to promote our own healing. Touch is an effective tool for triggering this natural healing response. Massage enables the body to relax, creating a therapeutic environment for the healing functions of the body.

The Stimulation of the Senses

Our greatest sense receptor, the skin, is the obvious target in **touch** therapies like massage, yet massage affects some of your other senses, too:

- The use of warm scented oil on skin activates the sense of **smell**, further promoting relaxation. If the oil also has medicinal properties, as is the case with many essential oils mixed within a plain carrier oil, the body's natural healing abilities are stimulated, helping the individual toward greater balance.

- Receiving massage with your eyes closed allows you to mentally visualize the soothing effects—**seeing** through feeling.
- **Hearing** soft calming music lulls us to an even deeper space of relaxation, allowing us to release all tension. The healing touch combined with gentle sound sends messages of trust to our brain, allowing the body to relax further.

Nerve and Tissue Response

Soft tissue responds to massage. The act of massage releases tension from tight muscles and supports the flow of oxygen throughout the body. As the circulation of oxygen and blood is stabilized, the body is encouraged to operate properly. Tight muscles can press on nerves and blood vessels, causing pain and reduced circulation. Massage helps to relax muscles, reducing these problems.

> ### The Purpose of Pain
>
> Pain is a natural signal alerting us to a malfunction within the body, an early warning not to be ignored. The pain response is present to sound the alarm, guiding us to seek the proper attention. Pain alerts us to begin the hunt to find the cause. Massage can be part of a holistic plan to eliminate pain.

Pain can have a negative effect on a person's quality of life and can slow recovery from injury. Massage can help reduce the pain from headaches, lower back pain, carpal tunnel syndrome symptoms, and more.

As the connective tissue of the body is restored to more efficient functionality through massage, pain is reduced. In addition, the emotional self responds with a deeper sense of well-being. This feeling of peace spreads to a spiritual level as massage sustains the connection of body, mind, and spirit.

What Does Massage Do?

Massage is able to maintain good health in various ways because it can:

- Create a relaxed state of being.
- Significantly reduce symptoms of stress, including anxiety and depression.
- Stimulate proper circulation, assisting the oxygen and blood to better flow through the body. Improper circulation can cause stiffness and muscle cramping. We all know what a toe or leg cramp feels like, especially in the middle of the night!
- Lessen headaches. As the muscles in the head, neck, and shoulders relax, an improved flow of oxygen and blood feeds the brain and surrounding nerves and muscles.
- Reduce chronic pain.
- Relax muscles.
- Increase immunity. According to studies in *The Journal of Alternative and Complementary Medicine*, massage therapy can help boost the immune system by increasing the activity level of the body's natural "killer T cells," which fight off viruses in our bodies.
- Boost mental health and wellness.
- Improve physical fitness. Massage can help reduce muscle tension, which can improve exercise performance and help prevent injuries.
- Encourage digestion and improve elimination.

Massage not only helps to maintain wellness, it also encourages the return of good health. Your body consists of many kinds of cells that make up the tissue of bone, skin, muscle, tendons, ligaments, and fascia, as well as nerves, veins, and arteries—all of which can experience pain and problems now and again, and all of which can benefit from massage.

Finally, massage is a complement to almost any medical treatment, further supporting the treatment's healing effects.

The History of Massage

Massage has roots in every ancient culture. People everywhere from the beginning of time instinctively touched others with kindness and love. To touch, to hold, to hug, to rub—these are inclinations that are universally owned. Even the earliest tribal cultures throughout the world included some form of massage when curing the sick. Tribal healers known as shamans served as priests as well as doctors, and physical healing was intertwined with spiritual healing. Early shamanic practice involved rubbing the skin as a form of healing. The shamanic technique was to rub the skin from the center of the body out to the extremities, ridding the body of the disease and bad spirits by pushing them out.

Eastern Massage Practices

The ancient Chinese developed the procedure of amma, or anmo, a massage technique of pressing and rubbing on specific areas to warm the extremities and heal the organs. Just as tribal cultures believed that body and spirit were not separate, so did the ancient Chinese, who believed if you heal one, you heal the other. Chinese massage was considered an important aspect of healing, and schools were developed to teach the different methods.

Anmo massage from China was practiced in Japan, and it eventually developed into shiatsu. Built on the concept of balance within, shiatsu was and is used to improve all functions by applying finger pressure along certain points in the body called energy meridians (see Chapter 18 for more about shiatsu and meridians).

Although the first written mention of massage is found in China, people traveled between China, India, and Egypt in the ancient world and research suggests that each of these regions may have developed a style of massage that is unique to their individual cultures. Some aspects are similar, however. India is credited with a form of massage and bathing known as shampooing, a massage method that is still used today in Indian and Arabic cultures. The massage techniques were done in a steam-bath environment, and the strokes included kneading, tapping, friction, and joint manipulation.

Massage in Greece and Rome

The practices of massage and exercise flourished within ancient Greek society. The physician and priest Asclepius was instrumental in the development of the famous Greek gymnasiums where the combination of massage, exercise, and water treatments were promoted to rid the body of disease and support whole health. Aesculapius was awarded the divine rank of god of medicine.

Hippocrates (c. 460–377 B.C.), known as the father of modern medicine, is also credited as a promoter of massage. Hippocrates's work was based on the idea that the body needs to be balanced to function properly. He prescribed massage as a tool to bring the body into wellness. Hippocrates revolutionized the practice of medicine with his new ideas and new procedures. He introduced the concept of symptoms as they related to the environment of the patient, using those symptoms as a guideline for treatment.

Hippocrates created a type of rubbing called anatripsis. The introduction of anatripsis revolutionized the practice of rubbing. Unlike the old shamanic style of massage, where the goal was to stroke toward the extremities to rub the evil spirits and illness out and away from the body, Hippocrates believed rubbing toward the heart to be more effective. He felt that massage moved the body fluids toward the center of the body, allowing for effective release of toxins and freeing waste to leave the body.

Even Caesar Got Massages!

Julius Caesar (100–44 B.C.), an epileptic, suffered also from neuralgia, a painful nerve condition that caused excruciating pain over areas of his body and head. He received friction-type massage as treatment for both the neuralgia and as a prevention of epileptic episodes.

The Roman era continued the support of massage and water therapy, using these treatment tools for chronic pain and muscle disorder, as well as for disease. Unlike the Greeks, the Romans instituted no formal training for physicians, and most doctors were undertrained slaves, barbers, or priests. Massage was often administered by slaves working in the gymnasiums. These massage providers could be called upon to practice medicine as well.

Claudius Galen (c. A.D. 129–216) was a prolific Greek writer and physician. Galen spent most of his years in Rome, where he provided massage and bath therapy to the gladiators as well as to a number of Roman emperors. Galen wrote detailed instructions for exercise, massage, and water therapy as treatments for specific injuries and ailments.

The decline of the Roman Empire brought unfortunate changes to the world of medicine, because many of the healthful practices were suppressed and forbidden. Although physicians and medical transcribers who lived through this long period of history still endorsed the use of massage, bathing, and exercise, these significant medical findings, along with other teachings, were nearly lost.

> ### What Is Allopathy?
>
> Modern medicine is built on allopathy, the use of drugs and surgeries to deal with the effects of the disease, but not the cause. Traditional medicine is homeopathic, meaning it treats the cause of the disease. Integration of the two styles gives you the best treatment.

Arab Physicians Keep Massage Alive

As Europe declined, the Arab nations endorsed and utilized the teachings of Hippocrates and Galen, as well as the ancient philosophers of Greece and Rome. A Persian named al-Razi (c. A.D. 864–930), also known as Rhazes, was a great Muslim physician and a productive writer who was greatly influenced by these early beliefs and traditions. This supreme clinician could describe the clinical signs of many illnesses. With this awareness he would often recommend the use of diet, exercise, baths, and massage.

Another Persian physician, Ibn Sina, also known as Avicenna (c. A.D. 980–1037), was heavily influenced by Roman and Greek medical practice. A copious writer, he is most famous for *The Canon of Medicine*. The *Canon* references massage and the use of baths and exercise as treatment of the classified diseases.

Massage During the Nineteenth Century

The natural treatment of disease using the ancient European healing concepts celebrated a renewal in the 1800s. Modern-day massage can trace its roots from this time period, when prevention of disease and the upkeep of good health became the goals of medicine. The revival of physical exercise as a form of natural healing can be seen in all aspects of healing work from this time forward. Drugs and surgery as methods for healing were in use, and some practitioners began to research the gymnasium experience as an alternative.

In the early 1800s, Peter Ling, a Swedish physiologist and fencing master, adapted a system of exercise known as medical gymnastics. Along with active exercise and active-passive movements performed with the help of a therapist, Ling's system stressed the importance of passive movements. These entailed stroking, kneading, rubbing, friction, gliding, shaking, and many more movements that are clearly massage techniques.

Ling established the Royal Gymnastic Central Institute, where the Swedish movements were studied. Schools flourished throughout Europe and training programs were developed to teach these healing techniques. Two American brothers, George and Charles Taylor, studied the Swedish movement and brought Ling's methods home to the United States, where they set up an orthopedic practice in New York.

Acceptance of the Terminology of Massage

Finally, in the late 1800s, the word *massage* was actually used to describe an individual healing component. Massage was considered its own modality with its own language. The terms *effleurage*, *petrissage*, *tapotement*, and *massage* were used when speaking of the application of these techniques in conjunction with physical therapy. Books were published, sharing instructions about Swedish massage as well as other information provided by physicians who used massage as a form of healing.

Massage Today

Today, massage is a viable profession that serves many purposes. A professional massage practitioner receives a structured training in a state-accredited school that teaches a detailed curriculum to prepare the massage therapist. Massage professionals have founded various organizations and associations that represent massage therapists and other bodyworkers as well. For example, the National Certification Board for Therapeutic Massage and Bodywork imposes strict standards of practice and requires continuing evidence of competency, bringing the status of massage into the realm of professionalism in healthcare. Most states now have a "Licensed Massage Therapist" designation for those practitioners that meet the requirements in each state. More and more communication is occurring between allied healthcare providers and highly trained and qualified massage therapists. Many hospitals now offer massage therapy within their buildings and in clinics.

Who Can Benefit from Massage?

Almost anyone can enjoy massage, as a giver or a receiver. It is the natural instinct of a parent to rub a baby's back. Doing so brings instant calmness and comfort to both the baby and the parent. We all reach out to touch another who is suffering from physical, emotional, or spiritual pain. A simple touch of the hand indicates empathy and compassion.

The specific use of massage can be found in many arenas and for all stages of our lives, including pregnancy, childbirth, elder care, and hospice. It is an important asset in healthcare today, and may be provided in chiropractors' offices, in physical therapy settings, in wellness clinics, and in hospitals as part of a patient's recovery plan. Massage is equally important in the field of exercise, helping the athlete stay fit and pain-free. The beauty business endorses the use of massage as well.

Massage and Recovery

Studies indicate compassionate touch speeds recovery from illness, and provides a release from tension that hastens healing. Whether a person is in the hospital or at home, gentle massage supports the return to health. As the tissues are massaged, the muscles relax and take in oxygen and blood, which helps the body gather strength. The depletion felt following an illness is often lessened, and at times even eliminated, through massage.

People afflicted with arthritis enjoy massage, finding relief from joint and connective tissue pain. Arthritis, a degenerative joint disease, is one of many in a group of diseases that share the commonality of inflammation, pain, and restricted movement of the joints. Massage provides one way to bring relief by allowing muscles to have better range of motion around the affected joints. Arthritis sufferers will often experience improved mobility and decreased pain with repeated massage.

> ### Don't Massage Inflamed Joints
>
> Joints that are inflamed from arthritis should not be massaged directly, though the nearby soft tissue and muscles can be massaged. The body is naturally protecting itself from further overuse by creating inflammation in those joints, which results in stiffness, swelling, excess heat in the affected area, as well as achiness. Wait until the swelling subsides before massaging the inflamed region.

Massage to Relieve Workplace Tension

Standing for eight-plus hours a day, whether as a waitress, a teacher, a builder, a nurse, or any other occupation that requires standing, puts great stress on the muscles of the back, legs, and neck. On the other hand, those who sit all day at their jobs might experience harmful stress to other joints and muscles, such as back, hips, and shoulders, which can inhibit natural circulation in the body. Frequent massage is essential for the health and well-being of all muscles when the body is stressed from constant standing or sitting.

Those who work with repetitive motion benefit from massage, too. Whether wielding a hammer or typing on a keyboard, constant use of the same muscles within the body structure can create chronic dysfunction in those muscles as well as the muscles in the surrounding area. People in service to others, such as medical professionals, emergency workers, educators, parents, and bodyworkers, call on their bodies to perform, often with no regard to rest. For those people, receiving massage is receiving instruction on relaxation. The person being worked on will surrender, and so restore the mind and the body to calmness.

Massage and Sports

Massage is a useful tool in the overall conditioning of muscles used for action in exercise. By stimulating muscles, massage tones them for peak performance. Massaging the muscles after strenuous exercise also helps to relax them, pulling out waste quickly. If an injury has been sustained, massage improves circulation and lymphatic function, allowing for speedier repair.

Don't Forget Your Pet

Animals love massage, too. Dogs and horses in particular will allow us to gently, yet firmly stroke with steady, even pressure along their muscles. A young pet learns to relax and receive, creating a pattern that can continue throughout the life of the animal. Cats, too, will allow massage, generally for a shorter period of time. Whatever pet you have, try gently stroking along the back or legs, introducing this form of touch slowly. Massage helps a nervous animal relax and creates an atmosphere of quiet tranquility.

Can I Learn Massage Myself?

Anyone can learn to massage—all it takes is the desire to learn how to provide compassionate touch. We all know how to touch with care; the next step is to discipline that knowledge into an effective system of massage. Massage is fun and it's also a source of pleasure and tenderness. Whether you massage yourself, a friend, or a loved one, the therapeutic art of massage brings awareness of the body to the forefront for you and the recipient.

Relaxation and Massage

The act of giving a massage is an instruction in total relaxation. Initial contact wordlessly educates the body to trust another and yourself so as to create an environment of healing. Every position silently focuses the recipient to let go, reminding the muscles to release, relax, and restore.

If you try the following simple exercise in muscle relaxation yourself, you can begin to experience the process of body awareness that is so important in massage.

1. Sit in a comfortable chair, your feet flat on the floor with your hands resting either on the arms of the chair or at your sides. If you prefer, lie flat on a mat, hands by your sides. Close your eyes and become comfortable with your breath.

2. Breathe in slowly, letting your breath fill deep into your stomach. Many of us do not use our lungs to their full capacity, rather we take short, shallow breaths. Inhale deeply through your nose, feeling the breath fill your diaphragm.

3. Hold your breath in for a count of three and gently exhale, feeling your abdomen contract, pushing the air out.

4. Inhale again, becoming aware of your hands; they may begin to tingle or feel heavy.

5. As you exhale, stay connected to your hands.

6. Once more, breathe in deeply and hold your breath, feeling your belly push out.

7. Slowly let the air leave you again, flattening your abdomen.

8. Gently shake your hands, feeling all tension begin to leave your body.

9. Relax your feet, letting each bone, muscle, tendon, and ligament relax and sink down to rest.

10. In your mind, move up to your calf and shin areas and relax them.

11. Feel your feet and lower legs become heavy, letting go of any hidden pockets of tension.

12. Bring your awareness to your knees; let them relax, sinking down into the ground. Feel your thighs and hamstrings relax.

13. Release the last remnants of tension from your hips and buttocks, letting yourself completely rest the lower part of your body.

14. Feel your back relax; let your spine sink down and relax; imagine every nerve and muscle in your back completely at rest.

15. Let your shoulders relax now and your arms; begin to feel every part of your hands from your wrist to your fingers; relax.

16. As you gently breathe in and out, every organ is relaxing, slowing down, as a sense of calmness permeates within; try to feel that calmness.

17. Now move up to your neck, letting all the muscles there relax.

18. Feel your face relax, your jaw, mouth, tongue, and teeth; let your cheeks relax as well as your sinuses and your nose; let your eyes and forehead relax.

19. Imagine a small glowing light appearing behind your eyelids, between your eye-

brows in the center of your forehead; this is your third eye, your psychic center.

20. Imagine this light and let it flow up to the top of your head and down the back of your body, following the spine and then the nerves, down to your soles. Color the light with a soft glow of pink or opal.

21. Feel yourself completely relaxed, every part of you free from tension and worry. This is the feeling we achieve when we experience massage. It is with this intention that we enter into a relationship with touch therapy.

Compassionate touch through massage heals on all levels. It helps us to relax, which in turn feeds the body, the mind, and the soul. It develops in us a sense of trust so that we can give massage as well as receive it. Giving and receiving massage develops a profound sense of self.

Chapter 2
The Importance of Touch

Babies and Touch

The first sense used in life is that of touch. Babies are cuddled, hugged, nursed, and wrapped in welcome upon entry into the world. For infants, touch not only signals safety, it triggers the growth hormone, giving them the go-ahead to grow. For children of all ages, normal metabolism depends on touch. Families live together in close quarters, sharing space, touching each other. This reassures children and adults alike that they are safe and all is well. We need to be touched to survive.

Touch not only encourages growth, it is an essential ingredient in the development of a well-adjusted being. Loving touch promotes spiritual, physical, mental, and emotional well-being. To be a happy, loving, intelligent, stable baby, child, and finally adult, constant tender caring touch is necessary. Babies begin touching while still carried inside their mother. Upon entering the world the first sense a baby demonstrates is the need to touch, whether by rooting about to nurse or grasping with little hands to feel his or her mother. There is no conscious thought involved, rather it is a driving instinct that allows the newborn to respond to the sense of touch.

How Does the Body Sense Touch?

The sensation of touch occurs because of receptors in the skin, known as mechanoreceptors. These receptors are capable of picking up three kinds (or levels) of sensations: touch, pressure, and vibration. Receptors are sense organs that receive information, known as stimulus, from outside or inside the body and then transmit this information as a nerve impulse to the brain, where it becomes feeling. Although conscious thought is not involved, the brain identifies the sensation and brings our awareness to the feeling.

The receptors that lie just below the top layer of skin respond to stimulation that, in turn, results in the sensation of touch. These touch receptors give you the ability to notice touch, whether it is light or discriminatory, described as followed:

- When experiencing a **light** touch, you recognize that something has touched the skin but you may not recognize exactly what is touching you or where. Feather-light touch that skims the surface of the skin creates a tingling sensation that remains even after the source of the touch has moved on.

- With a **discriminatory** touch, you know precisely where your body is being touched as the firm pressure of fingers and hands keeps you grounded in the moment. The touch receptors for pressure and vibration are found deeper in the body, in the lower levels of tissue. These sensations of pressure and vibration generally cover a broader area of the body and last longer than do the lighter touch sensations.

Temperature and Pain Receptors

The response to hot and cold is known as thermoreceptive sensation. Thermoreceptors are free nerve endings that respond to environmental temperatures, both internal and external. These receptors are found in the skin, the tissue, and the organs.

Pain receptors, known as nociceptors, are free nerve endings that are found most everywhere in the body, and are essential for survival. Pain is the reaction to overstimulation of the touch and temperature receptors. As these nociceptors respond to stimuli, they provide information and, if warranted, alert the body to trauma, letting you know that something is wrong.

Introducing Touch to Yourself and Others

Your skin can sense different levels of touch. You can recognize the light whisper of a soft breeze as well as the harsh pounding of ocean surf. You also have the ability to adapt to touch, such as when you initially feel the continued weight of your winter coat for a minute or two and then no longer recognize the added burden. The touch receptors in your skin become adjusted to the constant presence of the coat and so allow your awareness to shift elsewhere.

Touch as Communication

Touch is a form of communication. You gently touch your baby, rubbing her back, reminding her that you are here keeping her safe. You embrace your partner, then stay in close contact, letting your body brush slightly against his, keeping the connection. You greet a friend with a bear hug. You hold both hands in warm welcome as you connect with an honored peer or mentor. You may lightly touch the person you are speaking to, as a way of staying connected or punctuating the points of discussion. You meet someone for the first time, and you shake hands, briefly yet firmly.

Through each of these encounters, touch is the medium of communication. So much is said through touch, especially in massage where you communicate through different levels. The touch may be firm or deep. At times the interaction may be so light that it conveys the heat of energy without actually touching.

Talk, Then Touch

When massaging others, always gear the massage to the needs of the receiver at that particular time. Always communicate with your massage partner first to find out what areas he feels need some work. This strategy will help to create a comfort zone. Is the massage at the end of the day for relaxation or Ois the receiver returning to work and needs an energizing break? Find out if there are any chronically tight or painful areas. Ask the receiver if he is feeling anxious, under a great deal of stress, or has any particular areas that feel overworked or tense. The answers will lead to informed touch. Communicating verbally beforehand will help you better communicate through your touch during massage.

Using Your Intuition

Intuition is that part of you that lets you know where to work and what to do without any cues from the receiver. You may get an actual feeling, have a thought, or even see a picture in your mind of what will feel good to the recipient. Always listen to your intuitive self and be guided by what you feel, as well as what was talked about before you began your massage session. Touch through intuition adds depth to your massage, allowing you to be more than a technician.

Touching someone may trigger a response in your own body. For example, you may be massaging someone and feel a slight twinge of pain in your left shoulder. Using your body as a guide, you might massage the same shoulder on your receiver while gauging what strokes and pressure to use. Trust what you are feeling and you will likely find as you work that the pain in your shoulder, or wherever, will dissipate.

Touching with Compassion

Loving and compassionate touch creates an atmosphere conducive to self-healing. Caring about the well-being of the person you are working on allows you to give a massage to the best of your abilities. Wholeness of body, mind, and spirit is a concept you will be encouraging in all those you work with. Through touch, you allow a loving healing to take place. Your caring message can be conveyed to the receiver through touch. Kind touch says, "You are now in a safe place, you may release all tension and relax, totally."

> ### Palpation
>
> Palpation is an integral part of massage. Palpating means to touch the muscle tissue in order to gather information. You feel with your touch what your eyes do not see. You may not be able to see a dense area, but your fingers will tell you if the area has tight muscle fibers and is in need of massage to help it relax.

The touch of massage lets the recipient know it is the time to clear and cleanse, to let go of the toxins the body holds. The body welcomes release and is thankful for the compassion transmitted through the gentle touch of the giver. Muscles hold tension, which is a reaction to stress, and massage is a key method for relieving this condition. Often people push unresolved emotional issues deep inside, and the body expresses this tension.

Holding emotions in the body will cause parts of the body to tense up, essentially restricting the function of that part, whether it is a muscle, organ, or bone. As we lose contact with a part of the body, we generally reject that area, attracting overall dysfunction. A muscle will become tight, a bone may ache, and an organ will not realize its full capacity. Kind touch recognizes these rejected areas, and massage celebrates the entire body.

You can also help the receiver learn to rejoice in his body, to accept it as it is rather than how he would like it to be. Often the part of the body that is unappreciated or disliked will not function in the way the operator desires. The massage therapist teaches the receiver to experience the body as whole, even with its restrictions. Compassionate touch listens to the body and works to provide relaxation. Massage teaches the receiver to rejoice in the wholeness of the body.

Teaching Self-Love

Massage done with compassion creates an environment that encourages connection to self and approval of self. Self-criticism is held in the body as tension, resulting in painful muscles, achy bones, and congestion in the organs. Self-love releases these blockages and provides the balance necessary for wholeness. Understanding that distress indicates imbalance allows the receiver to begin a journey on the path to wellness.

Some conditions held in the body are chronic, meaning they are long-term conditions. Through compassion and love, massage can help those with such chronic health conditions learn to accept but not disregard them. You can help people to look at themselves as living with their condition, but not being limited by it. Embracing the concept of whole wellness allows people to choose holistic healing modalities, such as massage, that will help them live with chronic conditions yet not be ruled by them.

You can assist your receiver along his journey in healing. The compassionate touch you use helps the receiver to become focused on his body in love, and welcome recognition of it. Kind touch says, "I am worthy of love and I love my body the way it is." You can support the concept of self-love and appreciation by teaching the recipient to acknowledge the gift of life. The more a person accepts the body he lives in the more the body will change for the better. As a person grows to love his body, the body will work harder to honor its well-being.

When Massage Isn't a Great Idea

There are times when massage is not a good idea, because certain areas of the body are either too sensitive for massage or are inappropriate to touch. Use your common sense whenever you prepare to massage someone, and listen to what they are communicating. Certain underlying medical conditions may prevent you from giving or receiving a massage at a particular time. Also, massage is not a good idea if someone is in a lot of pain, even if you know the pain is due to a muscle spasm. We'll discuss this more in Chapter 4.

Ensuring an Appropriate Touch

Massage is all about the right touch. It is important to know when to use a certain stroke in massage, how much pressure to apply, and how long to stay in one area. It is equally as important to know when to work on an area and when not to. Always communicate with your receiver before a session so as to understand where the massage should be focused.

A feeling of well-being and inner calmness is the result of a healing massage. The contract between the giver and receiver recognizes the need of the receiver to feel completely at ease, confident in the ability of the giver to appropriately provide what is needed. You offer compassionate touch, together with respect and limit setting. The boundaries established in this sacred contract are workable and appropriate.

Areas of Sensitivity

Some areas of the body are best massaged with a feather touch or not at all. For example:

- Stay away from the area in the center of the throat because it is very sensitive.
- The neck area in general must be massaged gently, because nerves and arteries are close to the surface and very sensitive, too.
- Do not massage the eyes, or even around the soft eye area.
- Touch the ears very gently, staying away from the spot just under and behind the bottom of the ear.
- The arms have a few areas that you should touch softly: The armpit is very sensitive and often ticklish, so you may not be able to massage there. The inside upper arm, which is filled with nerves, should be massaged gently from the armpit down to the elbow. The elbow holds the "funny bone," a region that you know can cause a lot of pain if touched too hard. Not funny!
- The legs have a few parts that are sensitive, too. The inside of the top of the leg, where it connects to the pelvis is very sensitive, so do not press there too firmly because you can cut off the circulation, and it may hurt the receiver. The back of the knee should be massaged very gently. There are a lot of nerves in the lower edges of the ankle, below the anklebone, and in the back of the heel, so go softly there, too.
- The stomach is an especially touchy place—touch too gently and it feels ticklish; use too much pressure and it is painful. Ask the recipient how he or she feels about massage in the abdomen, and honor those instructions. Massage very steadily yet

gently and that should be just right. Some people may not like to be pushed and prodded in the stomach area, and that's okay, just move on.

- Lastly, the spine itself is not to be worked on; you can massage on either side but do not press on the spine.

Hostile Touch

Never, ever work on someone if you are angry with that person. Wait until you have discussed the issue that caused the feeling before you engage in any touch therapy. Because massage is a wonderful relaxant and instills a feeling of pleasure if done appropriately, touch should always convey the intent of unconditional giving, never anger.

If you are involved in a power struggle or conflict of any kind with the receiver, resolve the issue before you give the massage. Even anger not directed at your receiver may be felt, so wait until you feel better before actually giving a massage. Remember that massage is a physical and an energetic therapy, and what you feel will be transmitted through touch.

Genital Areas

Massage should never create a feeling of anxiety in the person receiving it. Always make your recipient feel safe. Make sure to drape areas that are not being worked on, especially the genital parts of the body. Leave no doubt in the recipient's mind that you are going to work appropriately. Through your confident touch and your no-nonsense manner the receiver will always feel safe and secure.

Light Touch

Whether you are giving or receiving, the quality of the touch is key to the enjoyment of the massage. Initially, contact should be light yet constant as an introduction into the energetic space of another person. You can place your hands lightly on the receiver's back, as this establishes a strong connection. Touching lightly yet firmly establishes the foundation for the healing environment.

The Effects of Light Touch

A smooth, light touch stirs memories from early childhood. Using light touch to design the safe environment of massage, you remind the receiver of soft blankets and loving arms. The recipient will sink down and relax, releasing the initial layer of tension as your light touch gives permission to let go.

Listen to the Receiver's Breathing

Relax your breathing so you can tune in to the breathing rhythm of the person on the massage table. See if the breathing pattern of the receiver is smooth and calm or if it is irregular and restricted. The rhythm of the breath lets you know how tense or relaxed your recipient is. Your soft touch is the signal to unwind, to let go of all troubles, to be still and calm.

Using Light Touch

The quality of your massage is expressed through your ability to provide consistent, easy touch. Place your hands lightly on the receiver to begin receiving information about that person's body. Use your hands and fingers to find areas of tension as you move easily across the receiving body, gently stroking it with soft, calming movements. Tension is recognized as tightness in the muscle, which makes the skin feel dense under your fingers. A shift in temperature from one part of the body to another can denote tension as well. Practice maintaining contact as you gently move your hands over the skin and muscles, assessing areas that are taut. You might also discover areas that are too relaxed.

What Atrophied Muscle Feels Like

A muscle that feels loose and flat indicates that the normal activity that creates the round firm shape of a healthy muscle is not being performed. An area that is too relaxed may signal the beginning of atrophy due to lack of use.

Deep Pressure

Light touch evolves into deep pressure as you move into the troubled areas of the body. Your hands act as your eyes, sensing where to work lightly and where to progress deeply, as your hands communicate to the body and the body communicates to you. When using deep pressure, be sure to maintain steady, sustained contact, touching to the core of the distress.

Applying Deep Pressure

Your hands and fingers are alert to finding areas that need deeper pressure, identifying knotted areas of tension. Shoulders and back muscles often require a deeper touch, once you have warmed up the body with light touch. As you move into these areas, feel the tightness under the skin. Slow, steady movement allows you to deepen the touch and effectively work the knots out.

Deep pressure is used to release areas of restricted circulation and to break up scar tissue. Scar tissue often forms adhesions and adversely affects the function of the area it is connected to. Adhesions are the result of tissues joining abnormally. They can be found anywhere, but especially around areas of dense, nonrelaxed tissue. These adhesions could be caused by surgery, after which they formed along the site of an incision. Adhesions can be released through deep massage.

Move Your Body

The best way to apply deep pressure is to move your body. Try this exercise. Put on your favorite reggae, hip-hop, or rock music and get ready to dance! Have someone lie on the massage table and place your hands on his or her upper back, with your body at the head of the table. Have your feet planted firmly on the ground, about a shoulder's width apart. Let your hands rest gently on the back and move side to side in time with the music; remember to bend your knees.

Notice how your hands begin to press into the back without any effort from you. Place one leg behind you, moving into a yoga-like warrior stance. Your hands will shift slightly; one may be a bit higher than the other. Keep moving in time with the music, and your hands will automatically press in deeper and deeper as you move rhythmically with the music.

Begin slow circular motions with your hands as you continue to move. As you move toward the table your fingertips will press in deeply. As you move away from the table the heels of your palms will apply the greater pressure.

Practice this type of moving on different parts of the receiver's body. Feel the rhythm rather than think about the movements. You are finding the groove that works for you, setting the memory of movement into your massage. Your body rhythm is far more effective than plain pressing with your hands. By using your entire body, the receiver feels deep pressure that is steady and assured. By employing your entire body, not just your hands and arms, you ensure that you can continue to perform massages for many years as no part of your body is overworked.

Keep Yourself Moving

Moving your body rhythmically allows you to apply deep pressure without pain to the receiver or you, the giver. Massage may generate a small amount of discomfort, what is termed "good pain," in the receiver. However, excessive pressure (causing real discomfort) will cause the muscles to tense up, creating injury. Remember to move, move, move!

The world of massage is a safe, comfortable place. Enjoy the feeling of giving as you receive. When you give a massage you are also getting. The pure joy of giving peace and comfort to another creates a sensation of peace and comfort in the giver as well. The magnificent world of touch awaits you.

Chapter 3
The Structure of the Human Body

Your Amazing Body

The human body is a fabulous, self-contained unit that functions in a state of perfect balance . . . most of the time. The various structures that make up the body communicate in a number of ways to keep their functions operating properly. The different structural levels ultimately group together into body systems that work together cooperatively; one system cannot operate without the combined efforts of every other system in the body. Having an understanding of these systems will help you learn the art of massage—when you know how the human body works, you are better able to restore balance when it is disrupted.

The Skeletal System

The skeletal system helps us move and protects our organs. It is composed of cartilage and bones that connect to and support the body. The skeleton contains 206 bones that are attached to the body by ligaments, tendons, and muscles. Bones work in conjunction with other parts of the body to keep us healthy. For example, bones store minerals and produce blood cells.

Your body continually replaces old bone tissue with new bone tissue. This perpetual replacement of bone tissue is called remodeling, and it continues throughout your entire life. Bones generally break down old bone in the center and form new bone from the outside. Along with the process of removal and replacement, remodeling places bones in the position of serving as the calcium storage unit for the body.

Calcium's Many Jobs

Calcium is necessary for many functions. For example, muscles need calcium (and magnesium) to perform the operation of contraction as well as releasing the contraction; nerve cells require calcium to perform the job of conduction; and bones need calcium to remain strong. Calcium is supplied to all the tissues of the body through the blood. The body constantly recycles the supply of calcium throughout the organs.

The Muscular System

The framework of the skeleton is moved by the contraction and relaxation of muscles. Your body is 50 percent muscle! Muscles make the body warm, keep the body stable, and see to it that your internal organs operate. There are more than 600 skeletal muscles in the body, all of which can benefit from massage, either directly or indirectly.

Types of Muscles

Muscle tissue is divided into three types: skeletal, cardiac, and smooth.

Skeletal Muscle

Skeletal muscles are also known as voluntary muscles because they move at your command. Skeletal muscles form the shape of the body and move the skeletal bones they are attached to.

> **What Is a Voluntary Movement?**
>
> Voluntary movements are those that you make happen by thinking. To walk, skip, run, or jump, your muscles are at your command. You can catch and throw a ball, type on a computer, turn pages of a book, drive a car, and dance all night because your skeletal muscles move voluntarily. Chewing food, smiling, talking, singing, or frowning are other examples of voluntary movements.

Cardiac Muscle

The heart muscle is known as the cardiac muscle. Cardiac muscle tissue is found only in the heart and provides the movement necessary for the heart to beat. This muscle is an involuntary muscle, meaning you have no control over whether or not your heart will beat. Cardiac muscle must be fed a constant supply of oxygen to support it. The muscle contracts and relaxes at an average rate of seventy-five times a minute.

Smooth Muscle

Smooth muscle is also an involuntary muscle, but this one is found inside organs, blood vessels, and at the point in the skin where hair follicles are attached. Smooth muscle tissue can stretch to a great length without losing its elasticity. For example, when the bladder or stomach is full, this muscle is able to stretch to accommodate the fullness. When the stomach or bladder is empty, the muscles return to their normal size, ready to be filled again.

Muscle Regrowth

The makeup of muscle fiber dictates whether or not it can regenerate. Some skeletal muscles have the ability to renew themselves and smooth muscles can regenerate considerably, but cardiac muscles cannot. Exercise increases the flow of blood and oxygen, which contributes to the growth, health, and renewal of skeletal muscles.

Functions of the Muscles

Muscles perform motion, maintain posture, and produce heat. They do this work through contractions that occur when an internal chemical process turns energy into movement. Some muscle motion is observable, such as running, dancing, talking, singing, and typing. Other motion you can't see, such as when you digest your food, when your heart beats, or when you eliminate waste. Your muscles sustain your posture by keeping you sitting or standing without falling over. Lastly, the contraction of muscles produces and maintains body heat. Think about how warm you get when you exercise; this is a perfect example of muscles at work.

Massage and Skeletal Muscle Tissue

Skeletal muscle is the type of muscle that is primarily affected by massage. This muscle consists of connective tissue, blood, and lymph, as well as nerve tissue. Blood and lymph supply food to the muscles and take away the waste. Nerves send the impulses for movement and sensation. Connective tissue makes up the bulk of the muscle and interconnects all the other body systems. Connective tissue is also referred to as fascia. You can think of fascia as a three-dimensional network of collagen fibers that surrounds and interpenetrates all the space within the human body from just under the skin on inward.

Massage works on the fascia and our many layers of muscle. Systematic and steady massaging of muscles makes us feel good and releases toxins that may be causing fatigue. Massage also helps to improve muscle tone, prevents muscle spasms, and improves overall muscle performance.

The Nervous System

The nervous system is one of the systems responsible for homeostasis; that is, keeping the body in balance. The nervous system responds to changes in the body through nerve impulses, adjusting body functions as needed. Homeostasis and whole health depend upon the proper operation of the nervous system, in cooperative partnership with the endocrine system.

The three main functions of the nervous system are to sense, respond, and integrate.

1. The **sensory** part of the nervous system monitors the stimuli that cause environmental changes inside and outside your body by checking with all your senses.
2. The **response** part monitors stimuli to your muscles or your glands. The integrative part analyzes the information received from the senses and assists in directing the motor response.
3. The **nervous** system is divided into two sections, the central nervous system (CNS) and the peripheral nervous system (PNS). The brain and the spinal cord make up the CNS, while the PNS is composed of the cranial and spinal nerves. The CNS interprets sensory information, sending out signals to muscles and glands as well as creating thoughts and emotions and storing memories. The PNS is responsible for sensory and motor impulses throughout the entire body, generating voluntary and involuntary responses.

Your Skin Is a Communication System

The PNS uses the sensory nerves to send messages to the brain, and it uses the motor nerves to conduct the messages from the brain out to the rest of the body. The skin is a main transmitter of both kinds of messages, receiving and giving information. As a result, massage is a valuable tool in stimulating or relaxing the nervous system.

Massage and the Nervous System

Massage affects the nerves, which in turn contributes to stimulation of most of the body functions. As the muscles and connective tissue relax, the nerves feeding all areas of the body seem to perform more efficiently. And as the nervous system functions at a higher level the body responds more effectively, reaching its highest potential. Good health is maintained through regular massage.

The Endocrine System

The endocrine system works in rhythm with the nervous system. The nervous system sends electrical messages to direct the body, while the endocrine system sends chemical messages. Endocrine glands secrete hormones into the bloodstream to keep the body in balance. Hormones from these glands are involved in your growth and development, and they are key to your reproductive process.

> **Exocrine Glands**
>
> Exocrine glands have ducts that transport the products of these glands into the body or onto the surface of the body. The exocrine glands are sweat glands, tear ducts, oil glands, digestive glands, and mucus glands.

Endocrine glands and organs containing endocrine tissues include the following:

- **Pituitary gland:** Secretes many hormones including those that control reproductive functions.
- **Pineal gland:** Produces the hormone that influences sleep patterns.
- **Thyroid gland:** Regulates metabolism, growth, and development, and the nervous system.
- **Parathyroid glands:** Help regulate the levels of calcium and other elements in the blood.
- **Thymus gland:** Helps produce cells that fight infection.

- **Suprarenal (adrenal) glands:** Secrete many hormones, including those that help the body deal with stress.
- **Pancreas:** Produces hormones that regulate blood sugar and help with digestion.
- **Ovaries:** Produce female sex hormones.
- **Testes:** Produce male sex hormones.

The Cardiovascular System

The heart, blood, and blood vessels are all part of the system known as the cardiovascular or circulatory system. The heart is a muscle that works constantly, twenty-four hours a day, beating sixty to eighty times a minute, pumping all the blood in your body through one full cycle, once every minute! Blood circulates through your body carrying oxygen and food through a system of blood vessels. A healthy heart can grow even stronger and healthier through exercise.

Blood Circulation

The heart has four chambers, known as the right and left atrium and the right and left ventricle. Blood travels through the body's veins and enters the right atrium. From there it is pumped into the right ventricle, and then into the lungs for oxygenation and removal of carbon dioxide and other wastes. The oxygenated blood then returns to the left atrium and passes down into the left ventricle. The left ventricle pumps the blood out to the rest of the body through arteries, where it eventually reaches tiny branches called capillaries. From there, the deoxygenated blood makes a return cycle through the veins and back to the heart. Valves in the heart stop the blood from flowing the wrong way.

Blood Pressure

Blood pressure is what forces the nutrients and oxygen into the cells of the body, which is why balanced blood pressure is important to good health. By maintaining a good level of pressure, the body keeps the blood vessels and heart healthy. Exercise, nutrition, and reduction of stress are all holistic ways to keep the heart functioning at its best. Massage is very effective in supporting the circulatory system, because it encourages the removal of waste and keeps oxygen moving through the body.

The Lymphatic System

The lymphatic system and the circulatory system work together. The lymphatic system consists of lymph, lymph nodes, lymph vessels, and lymphatic ducts. Lymph is a straw-colored fluid that is transported by blood vessels to fight infectious invasion to the body. The lymph nodes contain lymphocytes that help to remove bacteria from the lymphatic fluid before it reaches the blood. The lymph combined with the other organs of the immune system (thymus, spleen, and tonsils) hold the position of first guard in the body. Everything in this system flows toward the heart, continuously picking up waste along the way. Massage helps to keep the lymph system healthy, contributing to the body's ability to release toxins.

Breathing and Stress

Many of us live with chronic stress. Our bodies adapt to stress by developing habits to deal with excess stress chemicals. When we are in pain, or in chronic muscular tension, we tend to breathe in a shallower and faster way. This, in turn, can lead to chemical changes in the muscles and in the blood, further leading to stomach upset, headaches, muscle pain, cramps, or anxiety. Learning how to "breathe from the belly" and relax the chest and neck muscles can restore the better breathing habits you once had in childhood. As you give or receive massage, you can practice this kind of mindful, gentle breathing.

The Respiratory System

The upper respiratory system consists of the nose and the pharynx. Air enters through the nose, where it is warmed, moistened, and filtered. Hair in the nose filters out larger dust particles, while mucus traps the remaining dust. Small structures called cilia move the mucus and dust into the pharynx, which is the throat. From the pharynx, the mucus is either expelled or swallowed.

The lower respiratory system is made up of the larynx, trachea, bronchi, and lungs. The larynx is the structure that contains the vocal cords and is sometimes referred to as the voice box. The larynx allows air to pass to the trachea, or windpipe. The trachea flows into two structures, the right and left bronchi, which are air ducts that transport air to and from the lungs. The oxygen from the air in the lungs passes into the blood and flows through the body via hemoglobin, bringing nourishment to the cells. The waste matter in the form of carbon dioxide is moved out of the cells, into the blood, back into the lungs, and out of the body as we exhale. Oxygen remains in the body and the carbon dioxide is gone—the exchange of gases is complete.

The Digestive System

Food supplies nutrients that build and repair body tissues, and provides energy. The ability to nourish cells is realized through the chemical conversion of solid food to a usable form through the process of digestion. The digestive system comprises the organs that break down food into usable units: the pharynx (the throat), the esophagus (connects the throat to the stomach), the stomach, and the small and large intestines.

The digestive system also contains accessory organs that produce enzymes needed to digest food. The liver produces bile, which is used to break down fat in the body. The gallbladder stores bile until it is needed. The pancreas, a digestive gland that secretes enzymes to break down proteins, carbohydrates, and fats, sends these chemicals into the small intestine to assist the work of the stomach.

> **The Multitasking Liver**
>
> The liver has more than 500 functions. It is the largest gland in the body, producing bile to break down fat, storing important vitamins and minerals, as well as producing amino acids. The liver is the detoxifying gland, cleaning the body of such substances as drugs, alcohol, nicotine, and other toxic chemicals. The liver has the ability to repair itself.

The digestive system works to ingest, move, digest, absorb, and eliminate food. Ingestion of food is the process of eating. Movement of the food along the gastrointestinal tract occurs through a series of muscular contractions. Digestion of food involves chewing as well as the churning and mixing done in the intestines; once the mechanical process is complete, food continues to be digested through the addition of chemical enzymes. Absorption of food occurs when digested food is moved into cells throughout your body via the blood and lymph. Elimination occurs through excretion of the indigestible matter from the body.

Elimination of Waste

True elimination of waste involves many of the body's systems. For example:

- The respiratory system releases carbon dioxide, a major waste product from the cells.
- The skin allows waste to leave as you sweat.
- The digestive system removes waste through excretion.
- The urinary system keeps the body in homeostasis by removing waste and replenishing the blood.

The kidneys, along with the ureters, the bladder, and the urethra comprise the urinary system. These two small organs, the kidneys, also keep the balance of water, salt, and potassium in the body. (This function keeps you from retaining excess fluid, which can cause swelling in your hands, feet, legs, and other parts of your body.) The kidneys are also responsible for the production of urine, and the other organs either store or remove it. The kidneys also filter the blood, allowing nutrients in and keeping wastes out. All of the body's blood is cleaned and filtered by the kidneys every day. The ureters are responsible for carrying urine away from the kidneys to the bladder, where urine is stored. Once the bladder is full, the pressure of the volume allows the bladder to release the stored urine through the urethra, a tiny tube traveling from the bladder to the outside of the body.

The Integumentary System

The integumentary system is comprised of different but related tissue groups that combine to form an organ system that covers and protects the body. This system is comprised of skin, hair, nails, sweat and oil glands, and nerve endings. The skin is your largest sensory organ. Skin is your contact with the physical world, the vehicle for sensations of touching and being touched. Skin protects the body—it is the body's first defense. You even reflect your emotions through your skin, either by color, expression, or temperature. In massage, the primary focus is on the skin. Massage is a way to help keep the skin healthy, supple, and strong.

The Three Layers of Skin

The top layer of skin, the epidermis, is made up of five separate layers, which are responsible for things like protecting the skin and monitoring the passage of water. The epidermis also contains nerve endings for touch. The epithelial tissue that makes up the top layer of skin is continuously regenerating, reproducing cells that push up to the surface. As the cells move up through the layers they begin to die, eventually reaching the top layer of our skin, which then sheds the dead cells. The renewal process is continuous, and the rejuvenation of skin takes about three to six weeks.

What Causes a Tan?

Ultraviolet (UV) rays from the sun increase the growth of melanin, producing a tan. This process actually protects the skin from damaging radiation. Of course, too much exposure to these UV rays can lead to skin cancer. Moderate exposure to the sun and the use of sunscreen can ensure proper melanin production and help prevent the damaging effects of UV rays.

The cells responsible for pigmentation of the skin are also found in the epidermis. As new cells sprout from the basal layer (the deepest layer of the epidermis), some of these cells develop melanin granules. Cells called melanocytes produce the melanin that is responsible for the color of the skin. Everyone is born with the same number of melanocytes; it is the amount of melanin produced that determines skin color. Dark skin produces more melanin than light skin, giving extra protection from aging effects and environmental damage.

The second layer of skin, the dermis, is the layer that sits under and is connected to the epidermis. Blood vessels and additional nerve endings are found here, as well as the fibers that give skin its extensibility and elasticity. The dermis also contains hair follicles as well as sweat and oil glands.

> **Your Skin's Ability to Stretch**
>
> Extensibility is the capacity of the skin to stretch, such as during pregnancy, weight gain, or excessive swelling. Elasticity enables the skin to return to its original shape. At times the skin may stretch too much, causing tiny tears in the dermis that show up as stretch marks.

The third and deepest layer of the skin is the subcutaneous layer. This layer is made up of adipose tissue, which is fat, a necessary element to healthy skin. This layer of tissue connects the dermis to the bone and muscle beneath. The subcutaneous layer provides shape to the body and provides an extra cushion of protection for the skin above.

What Skin Does

The function of skin, actually of the entire integumentary system, is extensive. The skin is an efficient regulatory system that is essential to the maintenance of the entire body:

- It provides protection, produces vitamins, maintains and regulates body temperature, and removes toxic waste.
- It produces a protein called keratin that creates a waterproof shield along the surface of the skin, protecting the body from fluid loss and fluid gain.
- It serves as a line of defense against microorganisms and environmental invaders, such as bacteria, viruses, chemicals, and radiation.
- It acts as the first barricade against physical injury.

Types of Skin

Skin has many colors and textures due to many factors. Genetic makeup dictates some of the conditions of your skin, so do sun exposure, what you eat, whether or not you smoke, and other environmental factors.

Why Do We Get Wrinkles?

Wrinkles are evidence of early unprotected moments in the sun, although they show up on the skin in later years. Research has proven that people who stay out of the sun look six to ten years younger than those who are constantly sun exposed. Without a lifetime of sun exposure, your skin could remain supple and young looking until your seventies.

We have all seen ads that talk about different types of skin—too dry, too oily, or just right, whatever that might be! Actually, skin is an individual characteristic owned solely by you. Your skin is affected by your internal conditions such as hormone fluctuations, and by external conditions where you live, such as weather or sun exposure. Makeup, skin creams, skin cleansers, and any other type of skin care product also put demands on your skin. There are three main types of skin:

- **Oily skin** comes from an overproduction of sebum, which normally allows skin to be soft, smooth, and pliable. Blackheads are formed when pores are clogged by too much sebum.
- **Dry skin** is often caused by poor diet, environment, and age. Dry climate or winter air pulls much of the moisture out of our skin, leaving it taut and dry. With age comes dry skin, because the top layer of the epidermis is less able to hold water in.
- **Sensitive skin** can be the result of allergies, overexposure to chemicals, or too much sun. Cosmetics contain chemicals and fragrances that may cause sensitivity in some people. Most people develop some sensitive skin at some time in their lives.

The Effects of Massage on the Skin

The skin receives tremendous benefit from massage. Massage helps to remove the top layer of dead cells, improving the condition of the skin and making it look and feel healthier. Circulation is improved, bringing a new supply of blood to the sebaceous glands. As the fresh blood circulates, the sebaceous glands produce more sebum to keep the skin soft and supple. Improved circulation also stimulates the sweat glands, allowing for the release of toxins. At the same time the blood vessels expand, providing nutrients to the skin. Massage helps to release fatty tissue from the body as well as break up scar tissue.

Massage is essential to the support and function of the body systems. As massage reduces the stress in the body it allows the body and its various systems to function at the highest level possible. Massage is a preventative tool as well as a remedial benefit. Whether you have great health or are suffering from a chronic issue, massage is an important and helpful adjunct to better health.

Chapter 4
Getting Started

Preparing Yourself

Before you actually give a massage, you should allow yourself time to relax and de-stress. Remember, touch is a vehicle of communication; therefore, it is important to have calm, loving intention when you approach the recipient. Helping someone feel good is always a joyful event; the natural process of massage is an enjoyable way to spread the love.

Relax

There are many ways to generate and maintain a relaxed, caring attitude before giving someone a massage:

- Meditate or exercise.
- Give *yourself* a massage while listening to your favorite music.
- Try a guided visualization designed to relax you.
- Get out into nature and breathe deeply.

As you become familiar with various styles of relaxation, you will find those that fit you. The best forms of relaxation teach you how to listen to your body, and when you understand what you need, you can become aware of the needs of others.

A large part of massage work is tuning in to the person you are working on. If your massage partner has indicated that her neck hurts, then you know that is the area you will work on. But with experience, you'll also learn to listen with your hands. Perhaps when you place your hands on her shoulders, they will feel tight—clear indication that this area needs your care, too. Remember to relax and be calm as you approach the receiver. Let your hands become your eyes so that they may help you to discover what areas are in need.

Know Your Limits

It is essential to know that you cannot "fix" anyone with massage. Rather, you can use massage to assist or facilitate healing. Massage is a wonderful tool that can help us feel better, but if someone has unidentified pain you must send that person to a healthcare professional.

Stretch

Here is a routine you can use to stretch your body before beginning a massage. Stand tall with your shoulders relaxed and feet shoulder-width apart, with your arms hanging loosely at your sides. Close your eyes and inhale deeply, bringing your shoulders up to your ears. Exhale and push your shoulders down, feeling your neck stretch up. Repeat this three times.

Continue the relaxed stance and let your head fall gently to the right, remembering to breathe. On the inhalation bring your head up and gently drop it to the left as you exhale. Repeat this once more to the right and the left, then return to the original position with your head upright. Clasp your hands behind your back and step your right foot and leg out in front to a slightly bent knee posture. Stretch your arms away from your back; feel the muscles release. Bring your arms down, hands still clasped behind, and bring your right leg back in. Step your left leg out and, while bent at the knee, stretch your arms out in the back, hands still together.

Grounding Yourself

Be sure that your healing energy is contained within you and that you are firmly grounded. Imagine that your energy is flowing out from the bottom of your feet and traveling like tree roots deep into the core of the earth. Imagine a circle around you that keeps your energy within you, and a circle around the receiver that keeps her energy within her. Calm, gentle grounding can support a healing massage. Once you have achieved this grounded state, you are ready to begin.

Lastly, start by standing tall, reaching your arms up to the sky and joining your hands together above your head. Spread your legs slightly wider than shoulder-width apart and gently bend forward, scooping your belly in while reaching down with your hands. Stretch only as far as comfortable, bending your knees slightly. Come back up slowly to an easy standing position.

Consider the Receiver

Establish an opening routine in your massage practice that allows you a few minutes to discuss the needs of the receiver. Every person is an individual with requirements that are particular to her body, so it's important that you know those before you start. Listen to the issues that concern the receiver. What exactly is she looking for? Every massage should provide a relaxing experience, although some address specific problems: to help an ache feel better, or relieve a stiff muscle, or relax the whole body. Always check for restrictions in mobility and be aware of any chronic conditions that might prohibit a normal massage.

> **What Is a Chronic Condition?**
>
> Any long-term disease, such as diabetes or arthritis, is considered to be chronic because it is nonending. High blood pressure or thyroid disease represent other examples of long-term or chronic conditions. Something that will heal, like a broken leg or a poison ivy rash, is an acute condition.

Be Aware of Your Receiver's Needs

Remember that when deciding how to give each massage, you will be relying not only on what the individual is requesting but also on your own observations or line of questioning, such as:

- **How physically fit are you for your age?** Fitness level and age affect the choices you will have when administrating a massage.
- **Where are you going after this session?** What the receiver will be doing following the massage is another important piece of information.
- **Have you had surgery or injury? Where?** Find out if there are any previous or present injuries or surgeries; this will dictate your pressure and style.
- **Am I correct that we have one hour for our massage today?** Consider the time available for the massage. What are you able to accomplish in the time you both have allowed for this activity? Giving someone a massage late at night when you are tired is not such a great idea. A massage at lunch is fine, if you both have allowed enough time for what is needed. Beginning a massage just before the kids

come home for supper is not the best use of time. Plan to give massages when both you and the receiver have enough quiet time and space.

Arrange Your Space

It is also your responsibility to provide a quiet, private, clean environment for the massage. Prepare to devote this time to your receiver—turn off your phone! Whether you have an entire healing space or a beautiful screened area, the atmosphere must feel comfortable and protected for your recipient and for you. Take the time to create a warm, loving, secure space that is inviting as well as sheltered.

The rule of thumb when preparing for a massage is to make sure you and your space are neat and clean. Keep the space clear of clutter and free of dust. Set the tone with lighting and music to form a space that is inviting and restful.

Make the Receiver Comfortable

Once you have determined that you and your receiver are ready, make her as comfortable as possible. Use bolsters, wedges, and pillows; even rolled towels can provide extra comfort. Make sure you have enough sheets and blankets to cover the receiver so as to make her feel warm, safe, and secure.

Needs Your Receiver Might Mention

As discussed, massage is a useful tool in many ways for many situations. Here are some common goals you might encounter:

- Promote relaxation.
- Reduce pain, encourage healing, and reduce scar tissue and adhesions.
- Restore mobility, improve circulation, and aid in digestion and elimination.

The following information related to these common goals can help you approach your receiver properly.

Relaxing Tight Muscles

Massage can ease tight and stiff muscles as well as soothe muscle spasms caused by physical stress. In relaxing tense muscles, massage can also ease mental and emotional stress. Receiving massage helps the receiver make some positive change in body, mind, and spirit. Stress and repetitive motion are often the cause of tight, stiff muscles. Regular massage helps to prevent or alleviate symptoms of workplace positional stress.

Muscle Spasms 101

Properly functioning muscles are smooth with no discernable kinks. A spasm causes a kind of bump to appear along the muscle line, like a kink or knot in a rope. Stress on a muscle may cause these kinks to appear, interfering with proper muscle function. Poor diet or chronic dehydration can also contribute greatly to muscle spasms.

People who maintain certain postures all day in their jobs or who exercise often in a particular way may feel tight and stiff. Repeated lifting and pulling improperly can also create a pattern of pain or injury. Whatever the motion, if it is repeated often enough without proper care to form, muscle damage in the form of spasm or restriction of motion may result. Changing how we execute a task coupled with regular exercise and massage helps to prevent further injury and repair old problems.

Think about the stiff neck and shoulders that many people complain of, or the painful lower back and hips that prevent athletes from participating in events. These can be attributed to repetitive motion. Every action we take eventually becomes repetitive, simply by the act of living and aging. Massage can alleviate these painful symptoms.

Recovery from Injury

Once someone has sustained an injury, massage is helpful during the recovery period and beyond. Areas that have required stitches, once fully healed, benefit from massage to assist in preventing scar tissue and releasing adhesions. An adhesion is irregular fibrous tissue that results from an inflammatory process that starts during the healing of separated tissue, as in surgery or an injury. Adhesions can limit muscle movement by not allowing the fascia or connective tissue to respond to demands. Massage stimulates the fascial system, allowing the blood to flow effectively to all areas of the body, especially areas of injury. This nourishment helps the healing process, promoting skin and muscle health. The muscles become firmer and the skin becomes more supple with the application of massage.

When Massage Is Not Recommended

Massage is appropriate most of the time; however, there are conditions for which it is not beneficial and is actually contraindicated. *Contraindicated* means inadvisable. For some conditions, massage may be contraindicated entirely, while for others, only certain types of movements or strokes are not recommended. Contraindications in massage protect the giver as well as the receiver.

Some of these conditions deal with symptoms of a disease or particular physical defects, such as abnormal body temperature, inflammation, or vein abnormalities. Others deal with skin issues. Some are specific disorders and others are more general, though equally as important. Following is a rundown of situations where massage should be avoided.

Abnormal Body Temperature and Inflammation

If someone feels too hot or complains of being feverish, massage is not recommended. A fever is the body's way of fighting off attacks to the immune system. Generally, high temperature is a sign to let the body heal itself, without help from you at that moment.

Another reason for feeling heat might be inflammation in a particular area. You may be giving a massaging and find an area of the body that is noticeably hotter than anywhere else. Do not work on the hot spot because heat indicates an abnormality. Often such an area will have swelling and sometimes even discoloration. Advise this person to see a medical practitioner.

You might even see an open infection that is pus-filled or discolored. Pus is another way the body fights infection by localizing the infection to that area only. Massage could push the infection into the bloodstream, causing a more severe illness, so do not work on the person at all. This type of infection needs medical attention.

Vein Abnormalities

Following are a few conditions that affect the veins for which massage needs to be thoughtfully considered on or around the area affected.

Varicose Veins

Varicose veins are caused by the breakdown of the valves that allow blood to pass through the veins in one direction toward the heart. The valves act like inward opening doors, allowing blood to pass in only one direction, and keeping it from flowing backward. When valve action is faulty, blood flows back through the door, causing a bulge in the vein.

Varicose veins are usually bluish in color, greater than normal in size, and generally bulge out of the lower legs. Sometimes these protruding veins may be painful even without being touched. Varicose veins can be caused by prolonged periods of sitting or standing, when the valves may receive undue stress. Pregnancy and obesity may cause this vein condition as well. Varicose veins may also be an inherited condition. Varicosities can be found anywhere in the body, but occur most frequently in the legs and should be touched only with the consent of the receiver. When we work with someone who has varicose veins, techniques such as short upward strokes with plenty of massage oil can support venous return to the heart. Limiting the amount of friction to the area is also important, so be sure to use massage oil with gentle strokes.

Phlebitis

Phlebitis is an inflammation of a vein. It can be painful and is generally accompanied by swelling. Often phlebitis can evolve into thrombophlebitis, where a blood clot has formed along the wall of the vein. Massage directly onto the affected area is contraindicated if this condition exists. With consent from the receiver, start at a distance from the affected area with gentle, light strokes above or below. This can help to normalize peripheral tissues.

Broken Blood Vessels

When a blood vessel bursts, a small amount of blood leaks into the body. It is often visible just beneath the surface of the skin, as with a bruise. Broken blood vessels should not be massaged, but you can gently massage the area around the vessels.

Skin Conditions

Many skin conditions are *not* affected by massage. Your concern is with conditions that can be spread over the body of the receiver or to you. The rule of thumb is that if the skin is broken, cut, bleeding, or has a rash, do not massage. If the receiver has acne, boils, burns, blisters, eczema, or psoriasis, do not work on the affected area. You may massage other parts of the body, but not the affected areas.

Areas affected by sunburn are not to be massaged, nor should any parts of the body that have sustained insect stings or bites. If there is contact dermatitis or exposure to poison ivy, oak, or sumac, do not massage the body at this time, because doing so will spread the infection not only on the receiver but to you as well.

Muscle Cramping versus Spasms

When muscles are actively experiencing an intense spasm, which is greater than a muscle cramp, massage is not helpful. If someone is having such a powerful spasm that movement is close to impossible, suggest that person go to a professional massage therapist. Sometimes even a professional, however, will not work on the spasm and will instead make a referral to a medical practitioner.

Breathing Difficulties

Someone who has difficulty breathing should not be massaged. A person feeling disorientated, anxious, or panicky is not a candidate for massage, either.

Other Conditions

Some disorders require a doctor's go-ahead before you can massage. People on any long-term medication or medication for high blood pressure, asthma, nervous disorders, or cancer should check with their medical practitioners before beginning a session of massage. Individuals with these conditions can still respond well to massage, but a doctor's go-ahead is essential. Once medical consent is given, the massage should support whatever conventional treatment has been arranged. Advanced training is recommended prior to working with people with active cancer.

People with low blood pressure may feel lightheaded after a massage, so take care to allow someone with this issue to relax a bit longer on the massage table, and give a little extra assistance when the person gets up. Help her get up gradually: First have her sit up on the table and then look up. Next, have her put her feet on the floor, stand with her hands on her knees, gradually stand upright, and then walk forward.

People with heart disease can also do well with massage once their doctor gives the okay. Although these conditions and disorders do not completely rule out massage, great care must be exercised. If massage is allowed it must be performed gently, and the length of the massage should be reduced. When in doubt, do not massage.

Tools Used in Massage

There are a variety of ways to perform a massage. What you need is relatively simple: a flat surface, a private area, and most important, your hands. Once you have prepared yourself, and know the limitations of your massage partner, you are ready to organize your tools.

Your Hands

Your hands are your most valuable tools. To start, make sure your nails are cut short and straight across. Always check the length of your nails before beginning a massage. Use a good nail-cleansing brush to keep the nails free of debris and use an emery board to smooth out sharp edges.

Always make sure to cleanse your hands carefully with a good soap before you massage. You can use an antibacterial soap, but any soap will do; use what feels comfortable for your hands and your budget. Start with hot water, and soap both hands and forearms well. Rinse first with warm water, and then with cool water to close the pores. Wipe your hands dry with paper towels and dispose of the towels. Keep your hands moisturized, which will leave your skin smooth and less likely to chafe or crack.

Check your hands carefully for any open cuts. Be sure to look at the cuticles as well as the fingertips, and check over your forearms also. Do not work on anyone if you have open, uncovered wounds on your hands or arms. Keep a supply of bandages to cover all tiny cuts, and if you have any open, oozing sores, cuts, or skin disorders, do not work on anyone until these have healed.

If you are not sure your hands should perform massage, wait until you feel all areas in question have cleared up. However, if you feel strongly that you would like to massage a friend or family member you can always use rubber gloves. Keep a box handy if such an occasion should arise. You can also use a finger cot, which is a single finger of a glove, to use to protect a finger that may have a cut or open cuticle.

Massage Table

Next to your hands, a massage table is the most important tool you will use if you plan to give a lot of massages to your partner, friends, or family members. Working at a table is much more comfortable than kneeling on the floor over your receiver. Tables can be portable or stationary, but any table you decide on should be:

- Long enough to accommodate a tall person.
- Wide enough for the receiver's arms to rest easily on the table.
- Strong enough to support the massage receiver's weight as well as part of your weight as you lean in when working.
- Adjustable enough so that the giver can raise or lower the height safely and securely.

And make sure the table does not wobble!

> ### Massage Table Height
> Your massage table should be set at a comfortable height. To test this, place your hand flat on the top and keep your arm straight. Stand tall with both feet flat on the floor and relax your shoulder. If your hand rests easily, then this is a good table height for you.

Padding is important too; any massage table you use should have a good amount of thick, supportive padding to cushion the receiver's body. Several layers are best, because this will prevent the receiver from feeling the table and will provide a greater level of support. The idea is to allow the recipient to feel cushioned and supported at the same time.

You can find massage tables in stores as well as online. (See the resource section of this book for places to buy massage tables, such as Custom Craftworks and Costco.) It is easy to find a portable table, one that is strong, cushioned, and inexpensive. The beauty of owning a real massage table is the ability to provide massage in a safe and ergonomically healthy way. There are many good accessories to use with a quality massage table:

- A **face cradle** helps to keep the receiver's head and neck straight when lying facedown, while providing a space for the person to breathe. The face rest is made of foam and is fitted on a circular frame, which is attached to the end of the table. Some face cradles are adjustable, allowing even greater access to the neck. The cradle provides cushion to the face, support for the neck, and adds more length to the table.
- **Bolsters** are very useful to support body parts that need support. Bolsters can also be used to put the body in a neutral or gently stretched position. Be sure to place the bolster under the sheet so that it is not in direct contact with the receiver's skin.
- **Arm supports** can either add width or provide a shelf to rest arms. Side extensions can be attached to the sides of a quality massage table, giving more space for arms to rest slightly away from the body. An arm platform can be attached either to the face rest or to the end of a massage table. This shelf provides a comfortable place for people to rest their arms when they are lying facedown.

> **Keep Arms on the Table!**
>
> When lying facedown, arms that hang off the table may "fall asleep." You know, that pins and needles feeling! This means the nerve and blood supply is compromised. Whenever you are working on someone in this position make sure the person's arms are resting at his or her sides, or are supported on a shelf.

Regular Chair or Stool

You can also perform massages while the receiver sits in a chair. The receiver can sit on the chair, facing the back, resting the arms and head on the back of the chair. The receiver might even sit on a stool, with her head and arms resting on a table. The arms are folded with the head resting on the arms; usually a pillow is placed under the arms for support and cushion. When a receiver is in this position, you can easily work on the back and neck as well as the arms.

Massage Chair

A massage chair is a safer and more comfortable option. Such a chair can be simple to use and very portable. It is like a minitable, with a chest support, a headrest, and an armrest. Working with a chair gives you access only to the back, neck, and arms. Fortunately, these are often the areas people like to have massaged.

More on Bolsters for Support

Pillows, wedges, and circular bolsters are all supportive cushions that you will want to acquire. These will provide support whether the receiver is sitting in a chair or lying down. Here are some commonly used pillows:

- Neck cushions come in a variety of shapes, or you can make your own using rolled towels. Simply roll a bath towel into a tight cylinder, and slip it under the back of the neck. This will provide support and cushion while allowing the person's head to rest comfortably.
- A pillow placed under the knees helps to take pressure off the back when the person is lying face up.
- Facedown, a pillow under the ankles provides support and will prevent the feet from being in a position of "pointed toes."
- A wedge-shaped pillow is a versatile tool to place in the narrow edge under the knees, or under the ankles. A wedge can be slipped under the back as well.

Clean Linens

Acquire a good supply of cotton sheets that you use only for massage. Flannel sheets provide extra warmth and feel comforting in the cool months. White sheets are the easiest to keep in good condition because they can be bleached many times without appearing stained or discolored. Twin-size sheets are the perfect size. Be sure to cover all your pillows with clean pillowcases each time you give a massage. These should be cotton, too.

Bath sheet towels make great covers if they are large and soft. These provide effective coverage and can be used to drape around the receiver as he or she gets on and off the table. Towels usually can withstand being washed in bleach, too.

> **Keep Your Linens Clean**
>
> All sheets, towels, and pillowcases must be changed with each receiver. Never use the same linens! Wash everything in detergent and bleach, and then dry in a hot dryer. Wash massage linens separately; do not mix with your personal laundry.

Use lightweight yet warm blankets to provide extra warmth and cover. Fleece is an ideal weight for the cool months—it's easy to clean and very warm, yet not too heavy. A light cotton blanket or spread will work in the hotter months if extra cover is needed. All fabrics should be washable.

Soothing Music

Massage music can be purchased in many places. Any store that sells music will have a variety of relaxation CDs. Online music outlets such as Pandora, Spotify, or iTunes all offer a monthly fee subscription, and then you can conveniently play your music from your smartphone, computer, or iPad. Look for music that is instrumental, featuring soft healing sounds. Music for massage, yoga, meditation, and energy healing provides the soothing rhythm appropriate for bodywork. Some people prefer total silence, practicing in-the-moment mindfulness while they receive the massage. Always check to see what your recipient likes.

Gentle Lights

Natural light provides the best atmosphere for massage. If the room you work in has plenty of natural light, take advantage of it. Use curtains or blinds that allow the light to filter in while still providing privacy. Not all rooms where you massage will have the advantage of natural lighting. In such places, soft, clear lights work best. Use either small table lamps or a floor lamp placed away from the work area. Do not use harsh, glaring lamps or overhead lights.

Appropriate Draping

Privacy in massage is extremely important. It is essential that the receiver feels safe and secure. Let the receiver know that you recognize and respect his or her vulnerability, and that you are honored by his or her trust. It is easy to provide a secure cover; a flat twin sheet is very effective. Uncover only the part of the body you are working on; all else should be protected by the sheet. Be direct and deliberate when you are covering or uncovering a particular area to be worked on. Doing so is a very tangible way to protect the modesty of the receiver.

Let Your Receiver Decide

There are different stages of undress, depending upon the level of comfort the receiver feels. Let people know it is up to them whether they wish to be completely naked under the cover or if they prefer to keep their underwear on or even some of their clothes. The state of undress is a matter the individual should decide.

If the receiver is going to disrobe in the same room where you will be giving the massage, step out of the room to allow for privacy. Instruct the receiver to get under the nonfitted sheet in either facedown or face-up position. You may want to give the receiver a towel or robe to put on until you can help her onto the table. Some people will already be under the covers when you return; others may need your help. Of course, if you are working on your spouse or significant other, different rules apply!

Oils, Lotion, or Creams

Using a lubricant on the skin allows your hands to glide easily when performing the massage strokes. There are many different types of massage-appropriate lotions, each with a distinct purpose for use in a specific way. Experiment with a variety of products to find what you like best.

Whether you use oil or cream when you massage will depend on what you like as well as what the recipient prefers. Some people like the feel of a heavy cream sinking into their skin while others adore the feeling of warm oil as their skin drinks the healing properties. Some conditions respond better with the use of an essential oil applied in small, diluted quantities. Whatever you use, remember that what is most important is how good the massage and the products feel to the receiver.

> ## Ask Your Receiver
>
> Always check with your receiver to see if she has any known allergy or skin condition. Usually, the person will be aware of what products she can or cannot use. Discuss the contents of the massage medium before applying it. When in doubt use a hypoallergenic product, or ask the recipient to provide the lotion or oil she is able to use.

Using Oils

Oils provide a smooth, friction-free medium that allows you to easily massage large areas. There are many different types of oils: some are natural vegetable- and plant-based oils; others are essential oils; while others are made from nuts or seeds. Choose oils like these, because they nourish the skin. (Oils that contain alcohol or mineral oil, on the other hand, rob the skin of nutrients.)

Make sure you are aware of your receiver's tolerance to fragrance and nut-based products. A good basic oil is natural jojoba oil, which can be used alone or with essential oils. It does not spoil and generally does not cause any reactions. Another bonus is that jojoba will not stain the sheets or your clothing.

Using Creams and Lotions

Creams and lotions are thicker than oil and provide less gliding ability. Lotion absorbs easily into the skin, whereas cream needs more rubbing before the skin soaks it up. Both of these massage mediums are easy to use and are less greasy than many oils. Cream may be easier for you to use when you want to work deep in the muscle. Cream and lotion are both good to use on the face or any area where oil is not preferred. Cream also works well on regions that are hairy, like calves and backs, because the hands are able to glide easily and the cream keeps the areas moist.

Whatever you use to provide lubrication, always apply the medium to your hands first and then to the receiver's body. Do not put the oil, lotion, or cream directly on the body because the cool sensation will be jarring to the recipient. Be sure to rub the lotion into your hands to gently warm it first, and then apply it. You can have fun trying the different massage media, experimenting with everything, deciding what you like best, and practicing on yourself and others.

Lotion Warmers

Commercially available lotion bottle warmers can provide the recipient with a very relaxing and soothing experience. The bottle warmers maintain a steady temperature for the massage lotion or oil, and this warm sensation can be very comforting.

Chapter 5
Basic Massage Strokes

First Touch

You have prepared your space and yourself; now it is time to practice sensitive contact and learn how to enter the massage relationship with confidence and compassion. Your goal is to create an atmosphere of comfort and trust, conveying your sense of integrity and caring to the receiver. Your hands will become involved in healing as you practice and then perform different massage strokes on others and yourself.

The initial touch in massage sets the tone for continued relaxation. As with any touch therapy, it is essential to create an atmosphere of harmony that allows for total flow and release:

1. First, give the person receiving the massage a moment to relax as you become aware of the rhythm of his or her breath. Watch for steady, relaxed breathing as you approach the recipient.
2. Be sure the receiver is arranged comfortably on the table. Certain areas of the recipient's body may need added support, including knees, ankles, head, and neck. Remember, you can use a variety of pillows, towels, wedges, or bolsters to provide comfort and support during the session. Place these props under the knees or the head and neck if the person is lying face up; if the recipient is lying facedown, place a bolster under the ankles.
3. Draping with sheets is important for warmth and security, whether your receiver prefers to be clothed or not. Some recipients prefer to receive massage wearing underwear or athletic shorts and tops. Whatever a person feels comfortable with is correct for that person. You can use cotton or fleece blankets to provide additional warmth if needed.

Where to Start

There is no "right" place to begin a massage. Where to start on the body will become your choice as you grow into the art of applying massage. Some people like to begin on the back because it provides a large surface for the beginning strokes. Others prefer to start with a face or foot massage. Wherever you begin is the best starting point for you.

The back is always a safe area to begin because it is a nonthreatening zone with ample room to apply a variety of strokes, and it provides a broad canvas to begin relaxing your receiver. The following discussion explains how to use the back as your starting point.

Establish a Connection

With the receiver lying facedown, stand to the side, letting your body become comfortable with your position. Place both hands gently on the covered body, letting your still, quiet touch flow into the receiver. Let your hands rest in this peaceful position, encouraging deeper relaxation. This announcement of safe touch informs the recipient of the giver's intent. So begins your journey with informed touch.

As your hands gently rest on the recipient, breathe slowly and evenly, silently influencing the breathing of the receiver. Move one hand to the nape of the neck and the other to the small of the back, drawing an invisible energy line. Perhaps you would like to let both hands rest gently on the upper back, creating an energy connection there. The idea here is to allow yourself to become aware of your intuitive sense. Your hands are the tools that will guide you through this process, signaling areas where the receiver feels stress and discomfort.

What Is Intuition?

Intuition is defined as the act of knowing without rational thought. Our sense of intuition allows us to instinctively know or feel something without thinking and is an aspect of our senses that we use every day.

The first touch opens the pathway of communication between the body you are working on and your hands. See if you feel tension in the body under your hands. Is the back tight? How does the neck feel? Let the eyes within your hands reveal what the skin is relaying. Once you feel comfortable with your assessment, you are ready to begin.

Stroking Touch (Effleurage)

Stroking is the first general movement in massage. Stroking is just what it seems—long, defined moves that glide along the skin's surface. The technical name for this movement is effleurage (pronounced "ef-flu-rahj"). Effleurage is a smooth, gliding stroke that is employed in a variety of techniques.

Effleurage touch should be a light, soft movement as you begin to apply oil and soften the muscles. Your initial smooth gliding strokes allow you to cover a large area, introducing touch in a soft, acceptable style. Effleurage is applied using your hands, fingers, and at times your forearm. As you stroke the skin tissue you affect circulation and stimulate the lymphatic system. Once the recipient's muscles are relaxed, your touch should become deeper, pressing down into the areas of greatest resistance.

Effleurage strokes should be applied with lighter pressure as you move down the body and deeper pressure as you move up the body, imitating the flow of blood. By using lighter pressure going away from the heart and deeper pressure coming toward the heart you will assist in proper circulation throughout the body. By encouraging circulation, you help to clear toxins and supply nourishment to all the organs of the body.

Practicing Gentle Effleurage

Imagine the back as a clean canvas waiting for you to paint a picture. Stand behind the receiver's head, so that you are looking down along the recipient's back. Using the oil you and your receiver have selected, hold a small amount in your hands, letting the oil receive your body's warmth. Rub your hands together, coating them with oil, and place both hands on the back of the receiver between the shoulders. Move your hands simultaneously down the back on either side of the spine, spreading the oil.

Spinal Safety

Never press on the spine. If you gently run your fingers down the spine you will feel the bony vertebrae that protect the spinal cord. To avoid injury of this sensitive area, always work the area next to the spine, not on top of it. The muscles that attach to and support the spine are located next to the spine.

Keeping your hands on the back, move down near the waistline; then pull the hands back up toward the shoulders, still gliding. Continue to make long strokes down and long strokes back up, covering the entire back. It will seem as though you are drawing half-moons on the back. Let your body move in as you stroke downward and lean back as you pull up. Use a flat, open hand, keeping contact with the skin as much as possible. The strokes should continue to be smooth and gliding, eventually becoming deeper as the muscles begin to relax. Let yourself feel the skin responding to your touch. Each circuit around the back allows deeper pressure. Trust what your hands are telling you.

Fingers Can Be Used, Too

Some areas of the body are too small to accommodate your entire open hand when applying effleurage. When you massage the face, for example, use just your fingers to deliver long, sliding strokes. The fingers should gently glide along the surface of the face, bringing relaxation to a tense jaw or forehead.

The feather stroke is another form of effleurage. This involves letting the fingers act like fluttering feathers as you lightly stroke the surface of the body, using just your fingertips or your entire hand. Feathering gently calms the nerve endings, which is a great finishing touch to the part of the body you're working on. Gently feathering the fingers along the back is sometimes used as a transitional move from the back to another part of the body.

Kneading Strokes (Petrissage)

Kneading, or petrissage, is an effective technique to use after effleurage. Effleurage has softened the muscles, and now the body is prepared for you to go in deeper. In petrissage, you actually lift the skin and muscle, and apply a wringing, pinching, squeezing, rolling, or pressing movement. Simply put, it is a kneading movement that moves the deeper tissues of the body. This technique works to stretch the muscle, increase blood flow, and break up scar tissue.

Petrissage can be used over large areas of the body as well as on small sections. Use both hands on broad surfaces and one hand on smaller regions. At times only the palm or fingers and thumb are used, as illustrated in Figure 1, where the fingers and thumbs alone knead deeply into the back and shoulder muscles. As the grasped or pressed muscle is re-leased, firmly press on the area and move smoothly on to the next area in a circular motion.

Petrissage is an important technique, meaning that this is one to practice, practice, and practice. The rhythm of movement is important here. Remember to move not only your hands but your body as well, tailoring the amount of pressure by the rhythm of your motion.

An Exercise in Kneading

Practice the basic movement of kneading on the back of your massage partner. Stand to the right side of the body and place your hands on the left area of the back. Starting with the lower back, grasp a handful of flesh (the skin, fascia, and the muscle beneath it) in your left hand, lifting and squeezing without pinching. Use your entire hand with your fingers overlapping onto the flesh and your thumb a bit in front. Let your hand move in a circular motion.

Bring your right hand into play now, grasping another handful of flesh and repeating the same movement, holding the skin and muscle while moving the hand in a circular motion. Both hands should move in the same direction, firmly grasping the skin and moving in a slight circular motion. Move your body side to side as you perform this movement. Slide the flesh from your right hand toward your left and move your right hand up a bit along the back. The left hand grasps the flesh released by the right, and the right hand picks up a new section.

Practice on Dough

A good way to practice the kneading technique on your own is to knead some dough, either bread dough or play dough. Pay attention to how you must move your body in order to really see the dough change shape and texture. Practice all the different techniques of kneading while you work the dough.

Continue to roll, grasp, and pinch the flesh as you work up to the shoulder. Switch sides and work up the back again, using the same technique.

Remember to move your body in time with the motion of your hands. If your hands become tired, you may not be using your *body* to apply the pressure, which is where the effort should come from. Also, check to see how your hands are positioned on the recipient's body—if your wrists are bent, unbend them. If you tend to reach too far across the body, move your position so you are not off balance. Work up to longer stretches of kneading. Take breaks as needed until you strengthen the muscles in your hands. Your goal is to be able to perform this technique with no stress in your hand muscles.

Rolling Technique

Rolling is a kneading technique that uses the thumb and fingers to work only the top layers of tissue. Stay on the left side of the body, with your hands resting on the same side of the back. Your right hand is closest to the waist and your left hand next to it. Using your fingers and thumbs, grasp a small amount of skin and gently roll it back and forth. Your fingers push the skin toward your thumbs, and your thumbs roll the skin back to your fingers. Continue this back-and-forth movement as you move up along the left side of the spine to the shoulders. Return to the waist on this same side and roll up again. Repeat as many times as needed to cover this side of the back. Move over to the right side and repeat the rolling process there.

Wringing Technique

Wringing is a form of petrissage best used on the arms and legs. Imagine wringing out your favorite shirt—one hand twists one way and the other hand twists in the opposite direction. In massage, this alternate back-and-forth movement is gentle, yet deep. Use just enough oil to allow an easy, sliding motion as you wring up and down a limb.

Let's practice on the arms. It is easiest to apply this technique with the receiver lying face up. Help your recipient turn over by holding up the drape so that it hangs slightly away, letting him or her turn freely. Tuck the drape back in, leaving one arm uncovered. Standing to the side of the body, grasp the uncovered arm with both hands and firmly wring back and forth, moving up the arm from the elbow to the shoulder.

Bend the arm at the elbow, grasp under the wrist with both hands, and wring up and down the forearm. Use firm, steady pressure as you move toward the elbow, and a lighter touch as you move back toward the wrist. Finish at the elbow, wringing two or three more times. Rest the receiver's forearm on the table and cover this arm. Move to the other side and repeat.

Friction Strokes

Friction is a form of massage that moves the top layers of tissue over the deeper layers, causing the deeper muscle to be stimulated. Applied after effleurage and petrissage, this massage stroke allows the muscles to generate heat as they are rubbed together. Friction is good for releasing tight muscles, loosening scar tissue, and increasing circulation. Friction around joint areas reaches the underlying tissue effectively and may soothe aching joints. Use your fingers, the heels of your palms, and occasionally just your thumbs to apply friction, which can be fast paced or slow and deep. Generally the brisk style requires more oil, whereas the deeper movement needs very little lubricant.

> **Use the Appropriate Amount of Oil**
>
> If the movement is a gliding, sliding type of motion, make sure to use enough oil. Deep-tissue work, however, needs very little oil because too much may cause slipping from the area. Dry skin may need more oil, and so will elderly skin. Someone with a lot of body hair may need lotion and oil. Experiment!

The use of friction strokes in massage encourages the body to heal itself. The benefits of applying friction techniques are numerous. For example, friction techniques can:

- Stretch and soften fascia and connective tissue.
- Break up scar tissue.
- Increase heat in the body.
- Increase the local metabolic rate.
- Promote exchange of interstitial fluid (fluid between the cells and blood vessels).
- Increase circulation to skin.
- Increase circulation to joints.

Basic Friction Strokes

Ask your massage partner to return to the facedown position, and then tuck the drape in at the waist as you prepare again to work on the back. Stand at the head of the table looking down on the receiver's back. Taking a little bit of oil in your hands, rub your palms together and feel the heat from this small bit of friction. Place your hands on the shoulders, palms flat on the body, fingers close together. Lean in a bit and push your right hand down the back along the right edge of the spine. When this hand reaches the waist, push your left hand down along the left edge, while at the same time bringing your right hand back up to the shoulder.

> **Move Your Hands and Your Body**
>
> The movement of your body is essential to the success of your strokes. Remember to always move your body as you work with massage. Do not be afraid to move! Move back and forth or side to side depending upon the area you are working on and the technique you are employing.

Continue to work in this fashion, pressing one hand down as the other pulls back. Feel the heat under your hands as the friction begins to heat up the back muscles. Use your body to apply the pressure, creating a back-and-forth rhythm. This form of friction massage on the back moves in the direction of the muscle fibers.

Circular Friction

Circular friction is exactly what it sounds like—friction applied in a circular fashion. To practice this technique, position yourself at the head of the table. Let your hands rest palm down at the shoulders, fingers together pointing down toward the waist. Lift the palms of your hands up so your fingers are facing down with the pads resting on the back, then move your body forward and press in with your fingers.

> **Getting the Hang of Friction**
>
> To help you understand the feeling of friction, first work on a clothed body. With your hands on the receiver's back, apply a little pressure and circle on one spot with your fingertips. The shirt doesn't move, but the skin underneath does. This will simulate the feeling of one layer of skin moving beneath the other.

Feel the muscles underneath as they give in to the pressure. Let your fingers rest in the small groove or indentation you have created. Slowly begin to make small circles, moving the flesh, not the fingers, and feel the tissues under the skin move. Bring your fingers up a bit onto the surface of the skin and make circles again, with no pressure. Press in and cause friction. Feel the difference? When you apply pressure you are working the muscle and connective tissue (fascia) under the surface of the skin. When you let up on the pressure you are working only the top layer of the skin.

Cross Friction

Muscle fibers are formed in bundles of fibers that all run in the same direction. Cross-fiber strokes work across the muscle tissue rather than in the direction of the muscle fiber. This is a deeper movement for which you can use your fingers, thumbs, and sometimes the heels of your palms. Place your fingers on the area of stress, and move them in a walking manner across the area and back again. The pressure from your fingers causes the top layer of skin to move the under layer, without gliding, just as in the circular technique. Of course, most of the pressure comes from the movement of your body, as you move back and forth or side to side.

For deeper access, place one hand on top of the other while the bottom hand performs the crossing stroke. The palm should move across the skin with friction as the top hand applies more pressure. This technique allows for deep penetration to a painful area.

Tapping Strokes (Tapotement)

Tapotement, or tapping, is a percussive technique used to produce stimulation. The movement is a steady, even beat that produces a flush to the skin, a feeling of well-being, and a sensation of renewed energy. There are many different forms of tapping, and they are created by different positions of the hands and fingers. Some of the most popular forms are:

- Tapping
- Chopping
- Cupping

- Slapping
- Hacking

Keep Your Hands Loose

In tapotement, you always keep your hands relaxed. Practice for a moment. Relax your hands to keep them loose. Sit or stand and shake out your hands. Your hands and wrists will flap back and forth, your fingers will hit each other, and your thumbs will do their own thing. Let your arms fall to the side and relax from the shoulders. Allow everything to become loose and free.

Tapping

Next, practice tapping. Place your fingers on a hard surface, like a table, and start out slowly. Tap the table one finger at a time in progression, creating a smooth pattern. Let your fingers be easy and gentle as you move into a steady beat. You can use your thumbs to brace your hands as your fingers do the tapping. Pick up the pace; see how the table begins to talk back to you? When your fingers feel a slight pain, ease up the pressure but continue the beat.

Continue to experiment with tapping, making your own composition. The idea is to provide an even, comfortable experience for the receiver that will provide stimulation and add to the overall feeling of renewal. Tapping should not be so hard that it hurts! Rather than tapping harder, let the fingers all tap together; this will feel more intense.

Chopping

Let your hands form the chopping position, as illustrated in Figure 2. Let your fingers remain loose. Chop your hands slowly on to the receiver's thigh or calf muscles (not too hard or it will be painful) and pick up the pace as you become confident with this move.

Practice drumming and chopping on your legs so that you become comfortable with the feel.

Cupping and Slapping

Use an open palm with your fingers slightly cupped and gently slap your legs. Feel the slight vacuum caused by the curved palm. Now flatten your palm, straighten your fingers, and slap your legs. This feels different because the fingers do more of the slapping. Practice these two moves on your legs and find out what feels good and what is too much.

Hacking

Lastly, close your hands into very loose fists and pound lightly on your legs. This pounding or hacking is good for very large muscles such as those on the thighs or the back (but not near the waistline). Try this technique on yourself: Using your loosely closed fists, pound on your thighs with the sides of your hands; then turn your fists and rapidly beat a staccato rhythm on your thighs. Feel how the different ways of pounding stimulate your leg muscles? In massage, we call this hacking. This technique also works well on hamstring muscles, found on the back of the thighs, as demonstrated in Figure 3.

Become aware of the different feelings these tapping techniques deliver. After trying them all out on yourself, practice on your massage partner. Ask for feedback, continuously checking the comfort level of your receiver.

Other Basic Strokes

Vibrating, shaking, and rocking are massage techniques that produce relaxation or stimulation depending upon the delivery. These movements can produce a soothing effect to the nerve endings of the skin. Of the three, vibration is perhaps the most difficult to learn.

Massage with Vibration

When using a vibration stroke properly, your body will actually tremble. To get started, place your hand on your receiver's back. Bring your hand up so that only the fingers, mostly the fingertips, have contact on the skin. Let your entire arm shake from the fingers to the shoulder. Stiffen your muscles so that this shivering, trembling motion flows down into your fingertips. This is hard to do, so be patient. Once you have the trembling, shaking, shivering, vibrating movement under control, sustain the vibrations as you drag your fingertips, feeling the muscles underneath begin to loosen. The object of vibration is to free the muscles as you continue to move along the surface. Vibration and percussion can also be applied with massage tools such as the MyoBuddy.

Shaking the Muscles

Shaking helps to loosen tight muscles and helps to distract us from our habitual holding patterns. You can place your hand flat on a large muscle and gently shake the area. Or you can literally pick up an arm or leg and very gently shake it to free up tension. Lift the arm of your receiver straight out from the table and gently shake it, taking care not to pull or twist the arm. The muscles will loosen from the shoulder down to the fingertips. Another way to shake out an arm is to gently glide your fingers between your receiver's fingers, using your other hand to help you secure your fingers. You can also gently hold the receiver's wrist in your hand and shake carefully, as shown in Figure 4. Once the hand is securely held, you may stretch the arm up and out without any help from the receiver and shake it while your fingers are interlocked.

Another form of shaking is applied directly to the muscle. Place your hands on the receiver's back, using one hand to hold the back in place while the other does the work. With the working hand, shake the muscle underneath. This is a very subtle move, and you will need to pay attention.

Rocking the Body

Rocking is a fun technique that brings comfort to you and to the recipient. With the recipient lying on the table facedown, place one hand on the recipient's shoulder and the other on the waist. Gently begin to rock your body back and forth. As you do, your receiver will begin to rock also. Pull and push back and forth to establish your rhythm. Once you have a good rock going, the body will almost rock itself.

Experiment with rocking. As you rock the body, start to pick up a bit of speed. Once the body is rocking well, push but do not pull back, and let the body rock back on its own. An uptight body will resist rocking whereas a relaxed body will flow. Your goal is to create the natural ebb and flow from the rhythm of the receiver. Work with this technique for a while; try different speeds and different positions.

All of the strokes and techniques discussed in this chapter are the basic ones used in massage. Practice them and see what you like best. Experiment with how much oil or lotion to use, and find out which works best for you. Have fun and remember to move your body and exercise your hands!

Chapter 6
Applying the Strokes: Back

Working the Back

Once you and your receiver have prepared for the massage and the receiver is lying comfortably facedown on the massage surface, stand at the side of the table, place your hands on the receiver's covered back, and let your hands rest lightly on its flat, broad surface. Gently spread your hands over the back, as though pressing the covering free of wrinkles. Lean into the back using your body to create a rocking type of movement, letting your hands move down and up the back. The movement of your hands and the movement of your body create a subtle rhythm. Move to the head of the table and lean in with your body as your hands travel down the back toward the waist. Move backward a bit with your body and move your hands toward the shoulders.

> **Manage Your Oil Usage**
>
> Always make sure you have enough oil to move easily along the skin. The amount of oil you use should allow smooth, steady strokes on every part of the body. If you use too much oil, you will slip and slide, too little and you will limit your movement. Remember to spread the oil with gliding effleurage strokes.

Again at the side of the table, fold the cover and tuck it in around the receiver's hips. Apply oil to your hands and, with your hands flat, gently stroke down either side of the spine and back up again with long, gliding effleurage strokes. Figure 5 shows the proper position for your hands.

Remain at the receiver's head while you perform these effleurage movements six times. Next, move to the right side of the body and effleurage from the waist up to the shoulders and back down to the waist, applying more oil if needed. Your hands will push up along either side of the spine in strong sweeping strokes, then down along the outer back. Repeat these movements six times.

Now let your hands rest flat on the wings of the shoulder blades (the scapula). Both hands will be pointing in toward the spine. Move your hands in a circular motion over this area, on either side of the spine. Again use your body as you perform this technique, rocking toward the body and away as you complete the circles. Six circles usually will do.

Repeat this using your fingers, pressing in along the bony landmarks of the shoulder. Here you will make a smaller circular motion, actually resting one hand on top of the other and letting the weight of the resting hand move the tips of your fingers deeper, as shown in Figure 6.

Deep on the Shoulders

Move your hands up to the shoulders, bringing both hands to the left shoulder first. Using your fingers, stroke along the top edge of the shoulder blade from the spine out to the end of the shoulder. Actually press in with your fingers and gently pull toward your body off the shoulder. Stretch the skin in the same manner on the right side. Next, lay your hands to one side of the spine, pressing your fingers in as you pull down along the edge of the shoulder to the top of the arm. Repeat at least three times.

Deep effleurage in this manner along the entire top of the back, tracing the shoulder from the spine to the arm, pressing in with your palm and stretching. Continue to move down along the side of the spine, pressing in and stretching out every stroke to the edge of the body. Cover the entire back in this fashion, working on both sides of the spine. Stand on either the right or the left, depending upon which side is comfortable for you.

From the Side

Stand on either side of the body and let your arms reach across the back, resting your hands along the side of the back. This area is known as the oblique muscles. Using the kneading petrissage stroke, lift, roll, and gently squeeze along the entire side from the hip up to the under arm, as shown in Figure 7.

Be sure to assess the amount of pressure you are using as you lift and hold the skin. Repeat this movement back and forth along the side, eventually moving on to the back's surface. Continue to make imaginary lines from the hip up to the shoulder, steadily rolling and squeezing the skin until you reach the line of the spine. Switch sides and repeat. Both hands alternate lifting and kneading back and forth, following the pattern you have already established.

Pressing the Upper Shoulders

Move back to the head of the table and place both your palms in the nook of the receiver's shoulder just where it meets the neck. Press in with both palms, pushing and stretching along the top of the shoulder (the trapezius muscle) to the top of the arm (the deltoid muscle). Repeat this three to six times, pressing in firmly as you push down and stretch to the side. Check with the receiver to make sure the pressure is appropriate.

Using the Forearm

While still at the head of the table, move toward the receiver's right shoulder. Place your bent forearm on the receiver's back. Your elbow should rest alongside the spine, as shown in Figure 8.

Gently move the forearm down the right side of the back in a long sweeping motion. Using the forearm allows a deeper, longer stroke, covering a broader area. Move your body in as you glide along. When you reach just above the buttocks, known as the gluteal muscles, glide back up again. Continue for three or four times. Then move to the left side and repeat.

Do not use your elbow to press in, because this can cause discomfort to the receiver. Also you do not need to press hard; the motion of your arm and the movement of your body allow deep penetration without a lot of effort. Remember to check the receiver's comfort level.

Gliding Strokes

Place your hands flat on the left side of the spine near the base. Gently stroke up to the shoulder and back down to the tops of the buttocks. Use long sweeping strokes as you lean into the body. You are smoothing out the back muscles, so you want to use gentle, firm touch to encourage the muscles to relax. Move to the right side of the body and again effleurage down along the spine and up again. Remember, these are smooth, rhythmic strokes applied with the flat of your hand as you glide along the back. Glide your hands down and back in a half horseshoe type of movement on each side of the back. Coordinate your breath with a slow inhale as you glide upward and an exhale as you glide downward along the back muscles.

The Neck and Back of the Arms

Where you finish on the back suggests the transition you will make to either the neck or the back of the arms. If you are standing in front of the head, the logical movement is to the neck; whereas, if you end standing at the side of the body you will probably begin with the arms. This time you ended by the head, so you will continue on with the neck.

Neck

Start at the base of the neck. Using your finger pads, make tiny circles up into the base of the skull. You do not work on the bony spine region, of course. Small squiggly movements can be made up and down the neck using very light pressure.

Circle the entire back of the neck and then move up into the space on either side of the skull base. This is known as the occipital area, and it is covered by a group of muscles called the suboccipitals. Hold your fingers in at the notches just under the base of the skull right below the ears (to the right and left of the spinal cord). Pull in slightly, and you will feel the muscles relax with the easy stretch you are applying. This area holds a great amount of tension, so do not be afraid to press and hold firmly to the count of five.

Lastly, bring your fingers down to the side of the neck. Using a slight pinch and roll motion, move up the side of the neck and return into the occipitals. Press down and away along the ridge of the neck to the shoulders in transition to massaging the arms.

Arms

To begin massaging the arms, stand on the right side of the body with both hands resting near the top of the arm. Rest your left hand on the receiver's shoulder blade and your right hand on the deltoid area. Glide both hands downward in a smooth holding motion all the way to the hand. Repeat this three times from the shoulder to the fingertips.

Next, wring along the entire arm from the shoulder to the wrist; repeat this three times, down the arm and up again. Now lift the muscles of the upper arm and knead with a lift, pinch, roll movement starting at the shoulder and moving to the wrist. At the elbow, carefully and gently let your thumb and index finger make gentle circles around the bone, passing on to the forearm. Continue to knead with the lift, pinch, and roll motion, using your thumb and index finger as shown in Figure 9.

Gently pass your hand along the entire arm three times from shoulder to wrist. Repeat these moves on the other side.

The Lower Body

You are now ready to move on to the lower body. With your receiver still lying facedown, tuck the cover around his or her shoulders to keep the upper body warm. Lift the cover from the right leg and tuck the cover inward under the inside of the right leg.

Apply oil to your hands and starting at the right buttock use both hands to make smooth gliding strokes down the leg, making sure the leg has enough oil. Move back and forth three or four times. With both hands, wring all along the leg from just below the buttock to the ankle and back up again, three or four times. Now, starting from the top of the thigh, with two hands lift and squeeze the skin down the entire leg and back, twice. You can see how to hold your hands in Figure 10.

Come up to the hip. Using the pads of your fingers circle over the entire buttock on this side, firmly. Your fingers are looking for sore areas, which the receiver may have already indicated; if not you will find them. Sore areas generally show resistance with tight muscles. This condition responds well to massage.

Don't forget the side of the hip. With your left hand at the side of the hip, alternate between palm and fingers in a deep circular movement. Work around the entire hip area up onto the back of the buttock as well. Circle and knead where possible to release muscle tension.

Careful Spots

The depression at the ankle and the area behind the knee are places to be careful. Both of these areas must be worked with a light touch. If the receiver has varicose veins, do not work directly on the veins; rather, massage carefully around the area, if at all.

The Lower Leg and Foot

Now stand by the receiver's feet. Lift the right foot with both your hands. Keeping the knee bent, cup the underside of the foot with your palms while your thumbs make circular motions on the sole. Slowly lower the foot, gliding your hands to the back of the calf. Use all your fingers to circle up to the knee. Gently circle around the back of the knee, but do not apply pressure.

Bring your hands back to the ankle, and very lightly circle around the ankle area; this is a sensitive spot that does not need a great amount of pressure. Using all your fingers press in across the entire calf area horizontally. Slowly walk and press your fingers across the entire calf using a kneading motion, and work your way up to the knee. After you have worked the calf area sideways, begin again at the ankle region and walk and press up the calf to the back of the knee using vertical lines.

Using all your fingers, press up the calf, alternating your hands in firm, short pressing strokes. Stroke gently to the back of the knee and up the thigh, right into the buttock. Repeat this move three times, starting just above the ankle and pressing the heel of your hands into the leg with the same alternate strokes.

Next, start at the buttock and work back down the leg, squeezing in a wringing motion. Upon reaching the ankle region wring up the leg and back down again.

Cover the right leg and move to the other leg. Repeat the steps for buttocks, hips, legs, and feet on the left side. Remember to work rhythmically and apply more oil if you need it. Continue to check with the recipient to assess the quality of your touch.

The Halfway Point

You are now halfway through the massage and on your way to the next half, which is the front of the recipient's body. In transition to the next phase, adjust the cover so your recipient is completely draped. Standing at the side of the table, place your hands on the recipient's shoulders, with your fingers pressing in slightly. Lift your hands up a bit using the lift as leverage for your pressing fingers. Using steady rhythm, press in two lines down the body, on either side of the spine. Continue pressing over the buttocks and down the back of the legs. Press over the heels and down the length of the soles to the toes. Just below the ball of each foot, at the root of the toes, press your fingers in and hold for a count of three. With the same pressing rhythm, move back up the entire body to the shoulders, following the same two imaginary lines. Repeat your pressing movements, starting at the shoulders, working back down the body, ending in the center of the soles.

Chapter 7
Applying the Strokes: Front

Turning Over

To complete your receiver's relaxation, you'll need to massage the front as well as the back. The muscles of the arms and upper chest are involved every time you lift, push, hold, or carry. For this reason, it should not be surprising to find a lot of tension in these areas. As well, the muscles in the front of the legs hold just as much tension as those in the back. Facial muscles also respond very well to massage.

After you have massaged the back half of the receiver's body, he will feel completely relaxed. Although the receiver might agree that the idea of continuing with the massage sounds good, he probably would rather not move. Your request to turn over might be greeted with groans of resistance, so treat this time carefully. Speak quietly and offer assistance if it is needed. Always hold up the cover to ensure continued privacy while your receiver turns over.

Ask how the receiver feels as he rolls over. Suggest that he be aware of the muscles you have just massaged, and that he check to see if turning over is easy or difficult. Ask if the recipient feels tense or is able to move effortlessly. If the recipient feels tightness, reassure him that sometimes the initial reaction to treating muscles is resistance. The reason is straightforward: You have just worked on a large group of muscles that may have been holding the body incorrectly, and you have changed the operation of these muscles, giving them a suggestion of how to work properly. Muscles have memory, so the old memory may try to assert itself, causing an achy feeling as the muscles work in a new way. Continued massage will sustain the suggestions you have initiated. In addition, encourage the recipient to drink plenty of water throughout the day to flush out any toxins released through massage; these toxins can also cause muscles to feel achy after the toxins are released.

Once the recipient has turned over, settle the cover over his body. Check now to see where bolsters, pillows, or rolled towels are needed. If you were using a face cradle attached to the front of the table, remove it so you have easy access to that end of the table. Some people like a pillow or two placed under their knees and calves to take pressure off their lower backs.

If the receiver can manage it, use nothing under the head, or just a small rolled towel under the neck. You want easy access to the neck and upper back, and sometimes a pillow gets in the way. However, remember that the comfort of your recipient is primary; if your receiver wants a pillow under the head, provide one. Let your receiver settle in, relaxing again as you check his comfort level once more.

Feet and Legs from the Front

Stand at the foot of the table. Rest your hands on the tops of the receiver's feet. Breathe gently for a moment, feeling the heat from your hands spread out over the receiver. Undrape the left leg by slightly raising the leg, and then tucking the cover back under the left leg from the inside of the thigh. Support the left foot with your left hand, while the fingers of the right hand gently stroke down the top of the foot from ankle to toes. Smooth and press from the toes to the ankle; pull back up and press down again. Look at Figure 11 to check your hand positions.

Now, let both hands rest with thumbs on top so that your hands are cupping the sole of the foot. With a steady circular motion make imaginary lines with your thumbs from the toes to the ankle and back to the toes. Cover the entire foot with these imaginary lines. Gently press your thumbs between bones, stimulating the tendons and muscles on the top surface of the foot.

Next, lower the foot to the table and place your hands on either side of the foot, gently shaking and rocking the foot side to side three times. Keeping your hands on either side of the foot, with the flat of your palms on the edges, rub the foot along the sides in a circular movement.

Shift the cover to the recipient's left leg and move to the right foot. Begin with your finger strokes at the ankle and repeat the same movements you performed on the left foot. Before you continue up the leg, cover the recipient's feet and wash your hands.

Moving Up the Front of the Legs

Place both your hands on the calf of the recipient's left leg, just above the ankle, and stroke up the leg with long, smooth strokes as shown in Figure 12.

Your hands rest on the surface of the leg, pressing and stroking up to the hip. As you move up the leg, use firm, steady pressure pressing toward the heart. Apply gliding strokes with a lighter touch as you work down to the ankle. Repeat this move three times making sure you press and stroke around the entire hip. Move your body along the side of the leg as you stroke up and back.

Next, work your way up the entire leg, using the circular kneading technique as shown in Figure 13.

Use the pads of your fingers as you circle and pull the muscles along the shin and thigh. Lay your hands flat, then lift up to your fingers as you circle and press forward. Continue this circle-press-forward motion up the leg to the area around the hip. Move your fingers in toward the inner side of the hipbone and then circle out, applying steady, even pressure. Check with your receiver to make sure you are not pressing too hard.

Petrissage the Upper Leg

Stand on the right side to work on the outside of the recipient's left thigh. Reach across with both hands to lift and knead the thigh. Figure 14 indicates where you should place your hands.

Hold the flesh of the thigh between your fingers while you knead along the entire outside of the upper leg. Return to just above the knee and repeat the movement up to the top of the leg, just below the cover. Knead and lift along the entire thigh surface using less pressure on the inside of the thigh.

Wring and Roll

Move to the left side of the recipient and grasp the left leg at the ankle with both hands. Place your hands so that your palms are resting on the outside of the leg and your fingers are on the inside. Wring up the entire length of the leg and back down, repeating twice. Now place one hand under the leg and one on top and make a rolling motion. Roll your hands up along the entire leg and back down. Do this at least twice.

Drape the left leg and move to the right leg. Raise up the right leg and tuck the cover back under the right thigh from the inside edge of the thigh. Repeat all steps on the right leg, remembering to apply oil as needed.

Massaging the Abdomen

The abdomen is an area where you need to be especially conscious of your receiver's comfort. Some people love to have their bellies massaged while others do not. If your recipient doesn't want you to massage this area, proceed to the chest and arms.

If you decide to massage the abdomen, first offer to drape the receiver, using a pillowcase or bath towel to cover the upper body of the receiver, whether it's a woman or man. Some might prefer to stay uncovered. Tuck the larger cover around the hips. Stand to the right side of the body for easy hand placement, and begin circling with large gliding strokes from right to left three times, covering the entire abdomen. Refer to Figure 15 to see where your hands begin in this move.

Next, knead this region from right to left three to five times. Then go back over the entire abdomen with small circles, pressing your fingers in deeply. Continue to massage again, using your entire hand to make deep gliding strokes, pulling across the abdomen in horizontal lines. Gently stretch the skin away from the center of the abdomen to the sides. Complete this part of the massage by resting your hands gently on the abdomen, allowing the heat from your hands to flow into the receiver. When finished, pull the large cover back up to the shoulders and gently remove the towel from under the drape.

> **Benefits of Abdominal Massage**
>
> The abdomen contains the organs of digestion and elimination. Massage of the abdominal area supports the functions of these organs and improves circulation to the muscles in this part of the body.

The Chest and Front of the Arms

As you prepare to massage the upper body, make sure the cover is tucked in under the armpits with the recipient's arms resting on top. Stand on the left side of the body and begin with the recipient's left arm. Apply oil with firm, long strokes up and down the arm with one hand, as shown in Figure 16. Use your other hand to support the arm as the receiver relaxes, allowing you to take over.

Bring both hands on top of the arm and wring the arm from the wrist to the shoulder and back again. Feel the arm relaxing as you wring back and forth three times.

Support the arm again while the palms and fingers of your working hand make deep circular strokes from the elbow up to the shoulder. Each time you reach the shoulder, feather down and off slightly. Finally, lift and knead the flesh of the arm from the wrist to the shoulder, actually picking up the skin and muscle. Most people find that this feels exceptionally good, but check with your receiver to make sure the deep kneading friction is all right for him or her.

The Elbow

Use one of your hands to steady the recipient's wrist. Then use the thumb and fingers of your other hand to work the small muscles of the elbow. Your thumb is on the inside of the elbow and your fingers are on the outside. Be very careful not to press too hard. Use small circular motions first with your thumb and then with your fingers, as illustrated in Figure 17.

Lastly, apply circle kneading around the entire elbow, including the bony areas. Use your fingers and work all around them. Do not press hard!

The Hands

Hold the recipient's left hand in your left hand and grasp one of the recipient's fingers with your right hand. Press your thumb down each finger as shown in Figure 18.

After you press with your thumb down each finger, use your thumb and index finger to press and roll between each finger on the muscular area between each finger. Turn the recipient's hand palm up and use both your thumbs to wring the palm. Wring up and down the hand three times before stretching across the palm with both your thumbs, also three times.

The Shoulder

Still on the left side, use both your hands to glide up the recipient's arm to the shoulder. At the shoulder, circle the entire area on the top of the arm, using deep kneading strokes. Slide your left hand under the shoulder blade, and with your right hand continue to knead along the top of the shoulder to the neck. Feel the muscles along the upper arm as you knead in deep circular motions.

Supporting with both your hands, extend the recipient's arm palm up, out from the side of the body and up toward the ear. Move the entire arm in circles. You can see what this movement looks like in Figure 19. Circle only as far as the arm is comfortable moving, so be sure to check with your receiver.

Repeat the massage on the right arm and shoulder before moving on to the chest.

The Chest

Make sure the cover is securely tucked beneath the recipient's armpits, particularly for a female recipient. Then, stand at the head of your receiver, placing both your hands just below the neck on the top surface of the chest. The fingers of each hand touch each other and your palms are resting away from the center. Gently press down on this area, using very little pressure.

Move to the side of the body, facing the receiver, and place your hands on one side of the chest. Use your fingers to gently circle across the chest with imaginary horizontal lines. The pressure should be steady but light. Repeat three times. After the last circle across, press both your hands on the upper chest surface and hold, to a count of five, then release.

Massaging the Back from the Front

Stand behind the recipient's head and to the left side with your hands palm up. Gently slide both your hands under the left side of the back, with your fingers pressing into the back. As you move your arms down under the body, bend your knees so you have better control of your pressure and your body. In this bent-knee stance, stop when your arms can reach no farther down the back. Keep the backs of your hands resting on the table and press your fingers slightly into the back. Slowly begin to move your arms back toward your body, pressing your fingers and pulling your arms as you move.

Your fingers will feel any tightness or congested areas as you pull back. Stop on an area of congestion and move your fingers in small circular motions, still pressing in with your fingers. Circle on an area three times and continue to pull back, eventually straightening your body as you pull your arms out from under the back. Go in again and repeat this stroke before moving to the other side, where you will apply the same technique.

The Neck

To massage the neck, begin by oiling along the top of the shoulders and up along the sides and back of the neck. Turn the head to one side as you gently stroke oil on the neck with one hand and hold the head with your other. Turn the head to the other side and glide oil on this side of the neck, again holding the head with your other hand. Turn the head forward and cradle the neck in both hands, exactly as in Figure 20. Your fingers are pressing in under the neck and your thumbs are at the sides of the neck.

Using circular motions press your fingers in and gently circle and knead the back of the neck. This is another area to treat with extreme sensitivity, so check with your receiver to see if he is still comfortable.

Now, turn the head to one side, using one hand to support the head, and circle along the side of the neck with the fingers of your other hand. Move from the top of the shoulders into the neck, kneading the entire area. Press your fingers in along the neck while working up to the occipital ridge (the bony ridge under the ear). Refer to Figure 21 for proper hand position.

At the occipital ridge press and hold to a count of five. Repeat this stroke three times. Then turn the head to the other side and repeat your circling and kneading on this side of the neck.

Now, cup both hands again under the back of the neck. Make sure the head is flat on the table and gently pull the head; this is a wonderful stretch of the neck. Hold this pull for the count of three and release, pressing your hands down and gliding along the tops of the shoulders. Repeat two more times.

Working the Face, Head, and Scalp

Stand at the end of the table and begin the face massage with both hands on the recipient's chin. Apply a pinching motion with your thumbs and index fingers from the center of the chin to the edge of the jaw and back. Repeat at least three times. Use the fingers of both hands and walk from the chin to under the mouth. Using your thumbs and fingertips, walk gently along the skin in lines from the jaw over the cheeks to the sides of the face. Then, use your thumb and fingertips to walk from the jaw upward between the mouth and nose.

Starting at the sides of the face along the jaw, use your thumbs and index fingers of both hands to pinch and roll as you knead up both cheeks. This is a wonderful technique for sagging, tired skin. As you knead up the sides of the face, the receiver will feel the blood returning to the skin tissue. In the same upward direction, use a circling friction motion with your fingers to further stimulate the muscles of the face.

Use circular strokes on the forehead with your thumbs, as in Figure 22.

As you finish the thumb circles on the forehead, stroke the entire face with both hands from the jaw up to the top of the forehead. Bring your hands right on to the scalp and, using your finger pads, circle the top and sides of the head. Place your hands under the head and circle here using the pressure of the recipient's head as the application of weight.

Rest your hands gently on the top of the head and feel the heat of your hands penetrate the receiver.

Ending the Massage

All good things come to an end, and finishing with your receiver's head is the end of your full body massage, at least for now. Close your session with a quiet, peaceful energy, which will allow the receiver to transition easily to the reality of his or her life beyond your massage area.

Stand at the head of your recipient, gently placing your hands on the shoulders. Breathe easily and quietly, transmitting a sense of peace and calm to the receiver. Press in gently yet firmly with your hands and hold. Feel the shoulders relax further as the receiver's body sinks into the table.

Very gently and smoothly, stroke down the arms and legs, right through the cover. The idea here is to tuck in the good feeling, instilling your receiver with a sense of quiet wholeness. Move down to the feet and gently rest your hands here. Again, breathe slowly and evenly as you quietly rest at the feet.

The experience of massage will last long after the receiver comes off the table. The energy of the environment you have created along with the relaxing service you have provided will remain for some time. Leave the recipient by quietly saying thank you. Go wash your hands, allowing for a few moments of complete quiet. If you can give the receiver three to five minutes of undisturbed rest, how grand!

When you return, let the receiver know that he should get up slowly, enjoying the moments of calmness. Ask if your help is needed, and if it is not, give the receiver privacy to dress and come out of the room. Offer water and ask the recipient to sit for a moment.

You have completed your first massage. The wonder of massage is that you can repeat it over and over again. What's more, your intention to help is felt every time you give a massage. But remember, receiving is as good as giving, so make sure you have someone who will practice on *you*. Massage is a wonderful gift. Welcome to this great world of touch.

Chapter 8

Understanding and Relieving Stress

Understanding Stress

To be alive is to experience stress. Stress challenges us and presents us with the stimulus we all need to live. Without the motivation of stress, we would not think and we certainly would not act. The rhythm of life flows from the essence that is stress.

Typically, people view stressors as threats to their peace and well-being, resulting in a reaction. Stressors generally cause people to worry, feel overloaded, respond with anger, or become depressed. The result is that they feel they must protect themselves from any real or perceived event, particularly if the event is out of their control. Does this sound familiar to you?

How you react to stress dictates whether or not you are *distressed*. Distress becomes disease, so the key to stress is learning how to deal with the forces of life with ease. To flow through life without effort, embracing every situation as a lesson and using the tools you discover, is a goal worth achieving. Massage is a tool that can help you learn to go with the flow.

Daily Stress

Every activity you do involves stress because stress is part of living. Your positive response to stress allows you to survive with gusto, taking in all that life has to offer. Your daily routine consists of activities you have adapted to—your body, mind, and emotions generally know what to expect and they become comfortable with the routine. So the stress of your day-to-day life flows fairly well, but suddenly—zap—something happens to change your routine, and that disruption becomes a stressor.

Changes Cause Stress

Any change, even a pleasant one, can cause stress. Going on vacation or changing jobs is a stress. However, a change that you control affects you in a different way from a change you don't control. If you lose your job or cannot afford a vacation, you will experience that stress much differently from the stress you feel when looking forward to a new job or a fun getaway.

Too much stress, even of your own choosing, can cause havoc. If you thrive on chaos and constant upheaval, eventually your lifestyle will catch up with you. Assuming too much responsibility, creating undue pressure, thriving on overstimulation will cause an eventual imbalance. One of the biggest challenges facing people today is how to achieve a state of balance when dealing with stress.

Recharge Your Body

Your body's stress response began because our ancestors needed to flee from danger and fight for food. Those stressors do not exist for us on such a primal level today. However, a stressful meeting or an emotional confrontation still creates a highly charged physical response in us. Our body's reaction is normal, because, unfortunately, evolution has not caught up with our need to adapt our fight-or-flight response to present-day realities. Therefore, we often stay at a highly charged level, with our bodies running "on high," because physically fleeing or fighting doesn't often solve our problems today. After a fight-or-flight response to stress, our bodies need physical exercise to burn off excess energy, and then our bodies need rest to replenish our energy. Massage is one of the tools to help the body release stress, recharge the body, and renew the feeling of well-being.

Distress and Disease

The mechanisms of the body are constantly working to deal with the daily stresses of living. Homeostasis (the process of keeping the body in balance) keeps the internal functions of the body within normal levels as all the body systems work together in rhythm. If, however, stress goes beyond the normal limits, certain changes are triggered within the body. The physical response to stress is created by a chain reaction involving the central nervous system, the brain, and the production of certain hormones that explode through the bloodstream in the fight-or-flight reaction.

Stress has been here since the inception of humankind, and we have responded to the threat of danger in exactly the same way throughout our history. The fact that the human race can deal with stress has been instrumental to our survival. Ancient humans were able to react properly due to the actual physiological response that stressors produce, and the fight-or-flight response saved their lives. If an animal attacked them or they encountered a natural catastrophe, the response from within their bodies aided in their survival.

Today, you still have that built-in lifesaver that gives you the extra strength you need to either stand and fight or run away with a tremendous burst of speed. Think of the stories of mothers lifting cars off babies or of untrained civilians rescuing people from peril. The excessive rush of strength we get in the face of danger is due to the powerful way our bodies react to stressful or threatening situations. These tales of unsung heroes, professional and accidental, illustrate the body's response to stress—the fast heartbeat, the elevated blood pressure, faster breathing, and an increase in muscle tension. The body is also designed to relax and de-stress after every incident of the fight-or-flight reaction. However, many people do not take the time or do not recognize the physiological and psychological need to wind down.

The Chemical Response to Relaxation

Deep relaxation of the brain produces homeostasis. As you relax, the body produces more chemicals that promote feelings of well-being, such as serotonin for mood control, dopamine for emotional response, and norepinephrine for dreaming. When these chemicals flow freely, all body systems function at their best and tension is released.

How the Mind Influences the Body

The connection between body and mind has long been established. Your thoughts influence your emotions, and your emotions influence your body, and a cycle of body, mind, and spirit evolves. Thinking is good—unless you obsess. Obsessive thinking becomes obsessive worrying and this results in ill health. To be healthy, you can help yourself by recognizing that you can reverse the way you respond to stress. By relaxing your body and your mind, you can control your reactions as well as change how you deal with stressors.

Your mind can make you sick, but your mind can also help you stay well. As you become aware of the effects of stress, you can learn how to redirect your thoughts and emotions to create an atmosphere that supports good health. You have the ability to create a healthy environment for yourself by learning to change the way you think. Your brain affects your entire being, so relax your brain and you will relax your body.

Your brain acts like the processor in a computer; it is the center of all ingoing and outgoing information. Every thought, feeling, sense, and function is controlled through the brain from messages carried back and forth via the spinal cord. Stress affects the operation of the brain directly through the activities of the hypothalamus and indirectly through the responses radiating from the body. You can help the brain function at its highest level by learning to relax. As the body learns to relax, the mind can also relax, stilling the senses and rejuvenating the body. The power of your mind can keep you healthy, and your body can help your mind accomplish this task.

The Effects of Stress on the Body

Today's society is fast paced, with the emphasis on fast and busy. Everyone seems to be in a huge hurry to do more, be more, and get more, and part of the way to achieve all this is to stay in a state of constant "up." The body's response to this stress is to become more—to think clearer, to function faster, to be stronger—all of this and not feel hungry! Many people are so used to operating at a high stress level that they do not want to come down. The initial feeling of sharp intelligence, quick wit, and tremendous endurance is exhilarating. For many, the thought of not performing at this seemingly peak level is not conceivable. Yet the long-term effects of constant stress can result in chronic illness.

Your Stress Response Is Only Meant to Be Short-Term

The human function curve is a concept developed by Dr. Peter Nixon, a cardiologist in London, to demonstrate the effects of long-term stress. Nixon showed that, initially, performance increases under stress; however, over the long term, fatigue introduces decline in performance and, finally, ill health and breakdown. He also showed that long-term stress produces unawareness in the performer as he or she begins to decline.

Digestion and Elimination

Long-term stress can result in a number of health issues. Stress can be held in any organ or muscle of the body, so if you have an area of weakness, that area becomes a target for stress. Your stomach, for one, cannot manage ongoing stress without damage: Ulcers and other digestive orders are clearly linked to stress. Many people experience low-grade stomach upset every day and attribute this condition to a "nervous" stomach. If your stomach feels like this, though, you might actually have long-term stress. Furthermore, many intestinal issues such as irritable bowel syndrome, inflammatory bowel, or colitis are aggravated by stress. The body's instinctive response to stress is to shut down or slow down the digestive and elimination functions, and this chronic stress can, henceforth, become a serious medical issue.

Stress and the Skin

One of the first places extended stress can be seen is in the skin. Your skin is visible and you can see how you look whenever you want—and the day that your skin breaks out can be a stress in and of itself! The chemical imbalances caused by stress can change the condition of your skin, your hair, and your nails. All can become dry and dull, reflecting the effects of stress. Dry skin and dandruff, as well as thin and cracked nails can also be a result of chronic stress. More severe skin conditions like acne, eczema, psoriasis, and even hives may come from or be worsened by stress.

Your Heart and Your Lungs

Stress and the long-term effects of stress affect your blood pressure and the rate of your heart beat. Constant stress on the heart muscle weakens its function. A weakened heart leads to a weakened circulatory system, which adds pressure on the lungs as well. If the lungs weaken, they are unable to bring enough oxygen into the body, which leads to the problem of how to release toxic waste. You can see how not dealing with stress creates a mess of the whole body!

Stress and Your Muscles

The tension that stress creates as it prepares you to fight or flee puts an incredible amount of pressure on your muscles. During time of great stress you are strong enough to defend yourself and are also able to run unbelievably fast—more so than you normally would be. However, a prolonged stay in this condition may lead to a weakening of these muscles via the creation of trigger points within them, and that can reduce your overall strength and endurance. With the weakening of the muscles comes pain, and chronic pain is debilitating.

Imagine a condition where you try to use your body—to walk, play with your child, take the trash out—and a tremendous pain runs through your hip, stopping you in your tracks. You drink some water and try again only to be hit with even more pain. You attempt to continue but your body will not let you. The next day you are fine, and you continue with your routine, only to be hit again a few days later, this time far worse than before.

To add insult to injury that night you can't sleep because of the pain. You take a few aspirin and hop into the shower, only to discover that now you hurt all over; even your skin hurts as the water hits it. This episode sends you to the doctor, who may or may not be aware of the painful intensity or encompassing scope of chronic pain syndrome. Let's hope your doctor is aware, because this pain is real; it is not in your head! People who suffer from burnout may experience this kind of pain, which is another side effect of stress.

Balance and Stress

The nervous system supports the immune system and the immune system supports balance in your body. Both of these systems work with the endocrine system to help keep your body and mind fine-tuned and in a constant state of homeostasis. Normal day-to-day living creates stress that these systems can deal with; however, a continued barrage of stress-related incidents that leave your head spinning affects the way your body fights off disease.

Keeping the mind, body, and spirit strong gives support to all the functions of the body. Massage and other forms of relaxation not only teach you to relax but strengthen your ability to stay healthy.

Muscle Release Through Massage

You want to reduce your stress, let go of your tension, and feel relaxed all at the same time, right? Well, massage provides all of this, allowing you to be in the moment with your body and free of any stressors. Massage heals and invigorates simultaneously. The different strokes are designed to enhance health while preventing an unhealthy response to stress.

Massage teaches you to relax, encouraging all the systems to be in balance. The manipulation of muscles and connective tissue releases congestion and helps to tone the body. The release of tension promotes physical well-being while removing memory of injury from the muscle. Yes, your muscles remember repetitive motions. When you have a massage you are giving the muscles a positive experience, which helps you feel good both mentally and physically.

What Is Muscle Memory?

Muscle memory is the concept that muscles remember what the mind has taught them. This is why it is difficult to change a poor habit such as slumping posture or holding your head at a tilt. When you hold yourself correctly, it will feel wrong because your muscles remember the old way.

The effects of massage deal with the body's stress response and promote a relaxation reaction. How? Massage:

- Improves circulation and lowers high blood pressure, which supports the heart.
- Helps with digestion, keeping that system functioning smoothly, too.
- Releases toxins that could lead to illness (through your lymphatic system).
- Encourages the immune system to function strongly.
- Triggers the production and release of endorphins, the feel-good hormones.

Just as important, compassionate touch speaks to the human need for good, caring touch. Regular massage is an essential tool, teaching people how to react to stress with a healthy and relaxed response. By relaxing the muscles, you release tension, which helps you to face many situations with inner strength and a new outlook.

Other Relaxation Techniques

Besides massage, you can try many other techniques that provide you with the tools to relax and rejuvenate. Each one helps to combat the adverse effects of prolonged stress, prevent illness, and promote health. These techniques recognize the person as a whole being: body, mind, emotions, and spirit. A person's emotional well-being is directly connected with physical health, and both are connected with the mind. There are a wide variety of ways that you can learn to manage your stress. It is a good idea to study a few and find what works for you. The following relaxation techniques can all be used in combination with a massage program to help maximize your own stress reduction.

> **Health Alert**
>
> If you are pregnant, have a medical condition, or exhibit a tendency toward allergic reactions, check with your medical practitioner as well as a clinical aromatherapist and a trained herbalist before you use any oils or herbs. Never take essential oils internally.

Space Management

The practice of feng shui, the Chinese tradition of configuring space to harmonize with the spiritual forces that inhabit it, suggests that you should rid yourself of clutter. Whether you know it or not, clutter causes stress. So, if you have large quantities of old magazines, clothes, home décor, and other possessions that you don't need, don't want, and keep thinking you might use one day, get rid of them! Have a yard sale or give your old good stuff to the Salvation Army, St. Vincent de Paul, or any other such nonprofit agency. If you've been holding on to broken items, thinking you will fix them someday, toss them out!

Once you begin to clear out the clutter, check in with yourself and see how you feel—great, right? If you clear out old things physically, you will clear out old things emotionally and mentally as well. Keep up the good work and happy clearing.

Aromatherapy

The smell of oranges—ahhh—might remind you of summer days with your family, or some other terrific memory. Some smells make us feel happy and some make us feel sad, while some release stress. Both aromatherapy and herbal teas have stress-releasing properties; essential oils often come from certain herbs that make healing teas.

Chamomile, which can be used in aromatherapy and as a tea, is an herb that reduces stress and promotes sleep. Rosemary, another herb that stimulates the nervous system, is produced as an oil for aromatherapy and as a tea.

Proper Nutrition

You are what you eat, and if you eat foods that are highly processed and low in nutritional value, you are stressing your body. Even certain "diets" can actually be bad for your body. Before you begin an eating plan, make sure that is exactly what you are doing—undertaking a *plan* that can become a lifestyle. You must do more than just start a diet. There are organizations and numerous books on good nutrition that can offer you some basic guidelines so that you can devise your own nutritionally sound style of eating.

The Perilous Junk Food Cycle

Junk food may be designed to taste good, but it gives a rush of energy that is followed by a resounding crash. To reclaim that energetic feeling, many junk food eaters continue to eat those foods, which are deficient in nutrients.

Eating can be fun as well as sensible. Create a meal plan full of fresh fruits and vegetables as well as salads. Pick foods for the vibrant colors they possess and arrange the food artistically. Choose organic foods, which are foods that are not treated with chemicals and hormones, substances that add to the stress level in your body. Organic grains, fish, meats, and poultry can help you to sustain a healthy body and mind.

Meditation

The principle concept of meditation is to release stress from your body by calming the central nervous system. As the central nervous system becomes calm, you learn to stay in the present moment, to be still with yourself in body, mind, and spirit. Meditation calms the body and the mind so that you can resolve the issues that cause you stress, be they anger, depression, pain, or fear.

There are many forms of meditation, and just as many books to tell you how to meditate. A good place to start is with prayer, one of the oldest forms of meditation and positive affirmation. Use prayers that are familiar to you and set aside a particular time of day to practice. The longer you practice, the calmer and happier you will feel.

You may move on from your familiar prayers to other meditations or stay with what you know; the important issue is to find what works for you and practice it. Even with a busy schedule, you can set aside five to ten minutes a day to calm your mind. Try early in the morning before you start your day or before you go to bed as the last part of your nighttime routine, whatever works. Be disciplined and you will benefit.

Exercise

Exercise helps to decrease the effects of stress in a number of ways. For example, exercise:

- Builds muscle.
- Improves your circulation.
- Rids your body of congestion caused by toxins.
- Helps you to deal with stress because it encourages your nervous and endocrine systems to produce the chemicals that counteract stress.

Remember the fight-or-flight stress response? Exercise replicates the fighting/fleeing and tells your body that you have done your job and that your body can return to normal. As you finish exercising, your body recognizes that the danger is over and the relaxation phase can begin.

The key to sticking with an exercise program is finding one that fits your lifestyle. If you like being at home, pick something that you can do without leaving the house. (There are many good exercise videos you can purchase or download from the Internet and follow along with at home, like yoga, Zumba, Pilates, or tai chi.) Of course there are plenty of exercise classes, too, if you prefer a group setting. A gym offers many options and most gyms have classes in many different types of exercise as well as personal trainers and massage therapists. And don't forget walking, which is free.

Once you make a choice, try working with a program for one month before deciding either you love it or you want to try something different. Mark dates on the calendar each week for one month, and schedule the days and times you will work out just like you schedule other appointments. Whatever you choose, be it one form or many, have fun, and if you can take a friend along, so much the better.

> ### Stick with Your Plan
> The deal with stress management and relaxation techniques is that you have to make a commitment to follow through, which means you have to enjoy the technique. Find one (or many) that resonate with you. If you don't like what you find here, fine; design your own technique—take what you do like and devise something that works for you.

Bodywork

Massage is only one of many types of bodywork to choose from, and any form of bodywork is a de-stressor. See Chapter 18 to read more about reflexology, Reiki, lomi-lomi, and other forms of bodywork and specialized massage techniques. Within the range of choices you will find something to your liking. The chief issue to consider when choosing bodywork is what exactly appeals to you, because that will dictate what you are willing to try.

Massage is a stress management tool that creates a healthy reaction to life. The very act of relaxing enough to receive a massage begins the act of releasing stress, and massage in itself can be a form of meditation. Caring and compassionate touch supports the mind, body, and spirit connection, creating an environment that is healthy and sympathetic. The joy of living replaces the strain of life's stress as you utilize some of the tools you have discovered. Enjoy every moment of being.

Chapter 9

Finding a Professional Therapist

All Therapists Are Not Created Equal

Receiving is as good as giving. You have been busy giving everyone you know a massage, and now that you have tasted the richness of giving, it is time to feel the joy of receiving. Once you know where to look, you will find many different places to receive a massage, and many types of people who give them. (Along the way you may find that you want to study to become a massage therapist yourself; if so, congratulations!)

You need to keep several things in mind when searching for your ideal therapist. You want to be sure the therapist is qualified and knows what he or she is doing. It is also important that you like the way that particular therapist works. The glowing recommendation of a friend is not enough—you may find that your personal preferences are quite different.

> **Beyond Certification**
>
> Membership in professional organizations indicates the therapist is dedicated and serious enough to be a member of a governing group that upholds certain standards and ethics. Also, additional postgraduate study indicates that this therapist loves the work and is continuously refining his or her skills. Two of the largest massage therapy organizations are American Massage Therapy Association (*www.amtamassage.org*) and Associated Bodywork & Massage Professionals (*www.abmp.com*).

Checking Credentials

At the minimum, a practicing massage therapist has completed a 500- to 800-hour program of study at an accredited massage school, participated in a clinical internship or study, passed a nationally standardized written exam, and maybe also worked as an apprentice before striking out on her or his own. Most states currently license massage therapists and the remainder are moving toward statewide regulation and licensing. Most states also require a minimum number of hours of training, passing an exam to demonstrate competency (for instance, passing the MBLEx), background checks, as well as a certain number of hours of continuing education to be able to renew the license every few years. The MBLEx is administered by the Federation of State Massage Therapy Boards and is taken by massage school graduates. Next, the therapist applies for a license to practice in the state where he or she lives. Once the therapist completes the requirements for state licensing, he or she can call herself a "licensed massage therapist (LMT)" and can very often work with other licensed allied healthcare providers as a certified professional practitioner of massage.

When you begin your search for the right massage therapist, find out how many hours of training the therapist completed, if there was a practical requirement, if the therapist is certified by the school he or she attended, and if the therapist is licensed. If your state requires licensure, this license should be posted on the wall along with the certification from the practitioner's school and any other postgraduate advanced training programs.

Personal Taste

A wall full of certificates might not ultimately convince you that someone is the best massage therapist for you. The deciding factor may be that the therapist has a cheerful disposition, as well as a diploma from an accredited massage school and a state license to practice massage. Let your personal preference be your guide. Go with what feels best for you, physically, emotionally, and spiritually.

Equally important is the therapist's philosophy of massage therapy and bodywork. A therapist's philosophy is the set of beliefs, values, and standards that guide his or her work. An accredited and licensed massage therapist agrees in writing to uphold a code of ethics as outlined by the major massage therapy organizations, and these ethics even are discussed in the MBLEx exam. The ethics of massage are straightforward and true: to treat everyone with compassion, honesty, and respect, and to uphold the professional guidelines within the scope of practice at all times. (To read the full Code of Ethics, visit *www.amtamassage.org/About-AMTA/Core-Documents/Code-of-Ethics.html.*) Talk to a potential therapist to get a sense of whether he or she upholds these values.

Choosing the Type of Treatment

What is the right treatment for you? The answer to this question may change every day, because you do different activities every day and the needs of your body can change. To assess what the best treatment is for you, begin with what you like. If your preference is for deep muscle massage, consider how your body feels today as you move and exercise. How do your neck, shoulders, and back feel? Are your muscles tight or fluid? Tight areas in the large muscle groups respond well to a deeper massage, but the muscles of your neck may need something different.

> **Honesty Is the Best Policy**
>
> When you answer your massage therapist's questions, be up front with your answers, especially when it comes to medical issues. Your massage practitioner will base your session on what he or she observes and on what you say. It is important to reveal honestly the state of your health and how you feel overall.

The right treatment for you is what feels good and what helps you to improve your feeling of well-being. Stay open to new things and rely on your therapist to help you decide on the best treatment.

Describe Your Day-to-Day Life

Discuss with the therapist how a day in your life typically runs, exploring your energy level, your physical strengths and shortcomings, as well as what you expect to gain from your treatment. Together you will decide if relaxation is the primary goal or if you seek relief from chronic pain, or a combination of these, which will call for a variety of treatment styles.

What Are You Looking For?

If releasing stress is a primary goal, the massage therapist will address your tense muscles as well as your inability to relax. As the therapist begins to massage, you will feel anxiety and depression begin to fade away. The more relaxed you become, the deeper the strokes will go, soothing you to the core. Deep massage work is not necessarily painful, because as the body releases tension, it opens up to change on a deep level without resistance. A good massage therapist understands this.

If you want more flexibility in your muscles and joints, then you should work with a massage professional who is qualified to work through a series of strokes and massage styles that will best provide what you want. As the restricted tissues are released, the therapist may work deeper or lighter depending upon what your body is saying. Whatever your needs, the sense of contentment and deep release from massage will leave you glowing.

Looking for the Right Place

You know what you are looking for in a therapist and you know what you need, so where do you look for a therapist? Massage therapy is offered in beauty salons, spas, department stores, at your gym, or maybe even at your office. Many massage therapists work at the offices of medical practitioners, such as pain management physicians, osteopaths, chiropractors, acupuncturists, and naturopaths. Where to go to get a massage is an individual decision; do some exploring to find which of these environments is right for you.

> **In-Home Massage**
>
> Some massage practitioners prefer to bring the table to you. If that's what you choose, then your job will be to create a comfortable workspace for the therapist so that you can receive your massage in a peaceful and serene setting. Let others in your household know that massage time is your sacred time.

Massage and the Beauty Business

Many beauty salons recognize that taking care of yourself through massage is just as much a form of support as taking good care of your hair and nails. You stay healthier and feel better when you look good, and salons provide that service. As the business of wellness becomes more inclusive, many beauty salons now offer spa treatments.

Massage As an Allied Health Profession

Many medical practitioners offer massage in their office. Your chiropractor knows that you will stay adjusted longer and receive the work easier if you have regular massages. Other medical practitioners may prescribe a specific type of massage, like trigger point therapy, as a form of relaxation and for pain relief. Still others recognize massage as a complement to whatever treatment they are providing.

Massage Clinics

Massage schools hold clinics for their students to practice on all types of bodies. Clinics cost less and provide a broad spectrum of choices for you, the consumer. With such a variety to choose from you can experience many different touches and techniques. Contact your local massage school to find out when the school holds its clinic.

> **Look for Massage School Days of Wellness**
>
> Many massage schools also sponsor days of wellness where you can attend and receive whatever services are offered on that day. Generally, a day of wellness is a community service program and operates by donation.

Massage in the Mainstream

With the growing acceptance of massage, don't be surprised if you find an opportunity for therapy in the middle of your daily routine. For example, maybe your favorite perfume counter sponsors a five-minute chair-massage demonstration right in front of the counter to promote the latest scent. Or perhaps you come across a permanent chair-massage booth at the airport where, for a dollar a minute, the therapist massages you while you wait for your plane. Perhaps every week your office offers fifteen minutes of chair massage for every employee. Stress is everywhere, and massage is here to help de-stress people on their way through life, so take advantage of these opportunities!

What to Expect

You found where you want to have your massage and made an appointment with the therapist you like. Today is your first appointment and you are wondering what will happen.

Your massage therapist will greet you and then ask you a series of questions. These questions will range from information about your name and phone number to your medical history, allergies, and whether or not you are taking medication. You may also be asked whether there are certain areas of your body that are painful and what your expectations are—what benefits do you expect to receive from the massage? These questions are important for helping the practitioner understand how to proceed, and if any extra precautions need to be taken. Always answer honestly.

Training in Massage Therapy

Out of the hundreds of hours of training a therapist receives, generally 50 percent of it is hands-on, while the other half is spent receiving massage. The philosophy is, to give a good massage, a therapist must know what a good massage feels like. Today, the education requirements for massage therapists also include gaining a profound understanding of how the body and mind work in harmony.

A massage professional is trained to be a keen observer and an excellent listener. Massage therapists are trained to know when to refer clients to a medical professional, and how their work complements other therapies that clients may be receiving. The commitment of massage professionals is to support the wellness model within their own lives as well as those of their clients. Massage therapists need to know how to communicate with other care providers, and often are required to maintain detailed notes on what areas they worked on and how you rated your pain or discomfort after a session.

> ### Basic Requirements
>
> Professional massage training throughout the world requires the student to complete high school (or its equivalent) before moving on to massage school. Without the foundation of these basic skills, a massage therapist would not be able to handle the requirements of advanced training in massage, its techniques, and the physiological responses of the body.

As you know by now, massage therapy is more than rubbing backs. And it is more than getting paid for helping people feel good. Massage therapy is a complement to every part of life, from birth to death and all that is between. Massage is holistic—working hands-on, therapists help heal mind and body by providing relaxation and relief from stress, pain relief, better circulation, and detoxification. Massage therapists are highly trained professionals who love their jobs and relish the comfort and relief they provide.

The Course of Study

The study to become a professional practitioner of massage includes courses in anatomy and physiology as they relate to massage, in pathology, and in health and safety. There is a course in business that generally covers making a business plan and preparing for entry into the world of professionalism. Universal precautions for the health and safety of the practitioner and the client are part of every massage program. Student therapists also study the ethics of behavior, which deal with how to interact professionally while adhering to a strict code of values and conduct. In addition, aspiring massage therapists learn clinical documentation as it pertains to the profession, and how to make professional assessments that allow them to provide the best service for their clients. Students of massage also study its history.

The National Massage Exam

Following school graduation, a postgraduate goal is to achieve the national standard by successfully completing the national massage exam, or the MBLEx. This exam is administered by the Federation of State Massage Therapy Boards (*www.fsmtb.org*). Massage therapists may also choose to become board certified in massage therapy. The board certification is administered by the National Certification Board for Therapeutic Massage and Bodywork, or the NCBTMB (*www.ncbtmb.org*). The profession of massage recognizes the growth in its industry and sets standards and qualifications, which are recognized in this examination process.

Studies in massage continue after graduation, with the therapist choosing to expand his or her knowledge and mastering techniques in other bodywork methods. There are hundreds of NCBTMB-accredited continuing education providers all over the country. Some of these advanced training programs offer their own certification, such as Certified Myofascial Trigger Point Therapist, Clinical Thai Bodywork Practitioner, and Certified Neuromuscular Therapist.

The field of massage and bodywork is expanding and becoming increasingly more accepted as a field of complementary medicine.

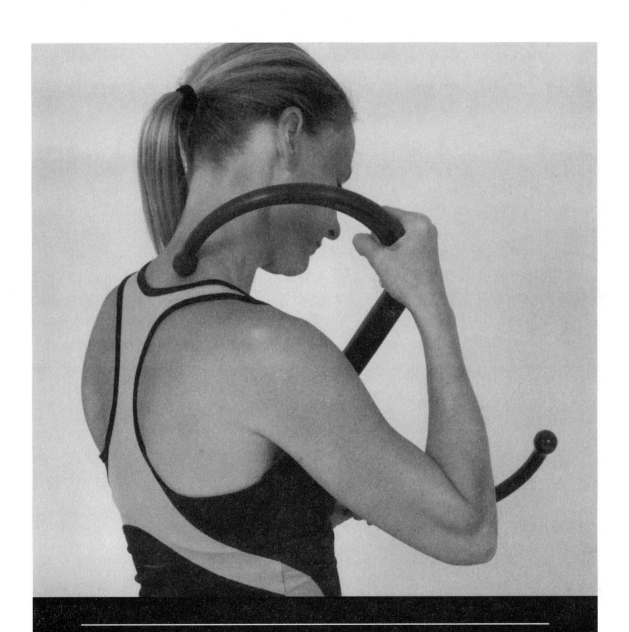

Part 2 **Special Situations**

Chapter 10
Self-Massage

Why Self-Massage?

To be a good massage practitioner, you need to know what the receiver feels. Practicing the techniques on yourself also gives you an understanding of how your touch feels to others. Performing massage strokes on yourself allows you to experience the effects of your own touch so that you may critique your own work.

Begin with Stretching and Breathing

The beauty of self-massage is you can do it anywhere. You can be clothed or not; you can be sitting, standing, or lying down. Begin with a stretch by clasping your fingers together as you stretch your arms out in front, palms facing each other, opening up your shoulders. Unclasp your hands and stretch your arms overhead, palms facing each other, as you gently rotate your head side to side. Stretch your torso from one side to the other, still reaching with your arms. Lastly, gently stretch your arms to the side, holding them out from your shoulders with your palms up. Let your arms come down to the sides of your body; you are ready to begin some mindful breathing exercises.

Safe Stretching

Know your body's limitations. When performing any stretching exercise, do not overdo it! Stretch in each direction within the framework of your own body. Adapt each maneuver, recognizing and embracing your comfort zone. Always listen to every signal your body sends you.

Rest both hands on your stomach area, one above the bellybutton and one below. Close your eyes for a moment and breathe. Feel your lungs expand and contract. Notice that your diaphragm is moving right below your rib cage. As you inhale, your abdomen expands and your belly pushes up. When you exhale, your belly contracts, helping to push the air up and out of your body. As your hands rise and fall with each breath, celebrate the cleansing your body is experiencing.

An Exercise in Silence

The ability to enjoy silence is truly a gift. To practice this art, pick a time when you know you will not be interrupted. Perhaps this means getting up fifteen minutes earlier than others in your household, or staying up fifteen minutes later. Maybe you work at home and you can take fifteen minutes to be alone sometime during your workday. If you are parenting a newborn or toddler, plan your silent time during baby's naptime.

> ### Be Kind to Yourself
>
> Many people feel that it is selfish to set aside personal time. However, it is not selfish to nourish yourself first; if you are not sustained, you cannot sustain anyone else. Selfishness means not sharing the gifts of your abundance, like not sharing extra food or clothing.

Cover yourself with a light blanket and sit or lie quietly, with your eyes closed and your palms resting face up. Breathe in slowly and fully, letting your breath fill your abdomen. Release your breath completely and continue to follow this pattern with slow, quiet breathing. Listen to your body as your heartbeat begins to speak. Relax into this rhythm.

Visualize yourself sitting or lying in a huge tub, relaxed, ready to receive. Picture someone you love approaching with a huge pitcher filled with a golden liquid; the word "love" floating on top of the fluid. As you rest, your partner pours endless amounts of golden love over you, washing you completely, allowing you to feel full of love. Relax and allow this feeling to flow through your body; notice how your belly may tickle with joy and your energy is calm. Become aware of your breathing again and slowly stretch, and open your eyes.

Massaging Your Abdomen

The abdomen is the center of your being. Many important organs are housed within this area of your body. In many traditional Eastern philosophies, the abdomen is known as the hara, the center of the life force.

Touching the center of yourself is to honor you. You don't have to take off your clothes, just sit or lie in a comfortable space. You can perform all the strokes without oil or lotion if you prefer. (Whether or not you use oil or lotion for this exercise will depend upon your state of dress or undress.) Place your hands gently on your abdomen, and feel the light touch. Relax as your hands press lightly on your body, creating a moment of quiet release. This is the holding stroke.

Rest one hand on your thigh while the other hand glides in a circle around your abdomen. Always start on your right side and move clockwise. The large intestine (the colon) begins just above your pubic bone on the right side of your body. It curves up the right side, across the waist to the left, and then down along the left side before reaching the rectum. Massage strokes support the function of the inner organs, therefore you work in the direction of movement. The colon is the last stop before excretion of solids from the body, so you massage in the direction of elimination. The gliding strokes support the process of movement, freeing toxins and relaxing the colon.

Surface kneading of the abdomen allows the blood to circulate, toning the skin. Using both hands, grasp the skin of your abdomen between your fingers and thumbs, lift up, pinch, and roll. Knead with both hands moving from below your belly up to your ribs and then down again. Bring your hands to the sides of your abdomen and knead in toward the center with the pinching, rolling motion. When your fingers meet, stretch and roll the skin back to your sides.

Bring both hands to the lower right section of your abdomen and knead deeply, using your fingers to press in before you lift, pinch, and roll. Move up along the right side to your rib cage, following the path of the ascending colon. Continue the motion across your waistline and down the left side turning in toward the lower center of your abdomen. Work with this press-lift-pinch-roll rhythm over your entire abdominal surface.

Don't Be Afraid of Gas

Working on the abdominopelvic region will release pockets of air from the small and large intestines. Belching and flatulence caused by excessive amounts of air in the stomach or intestines may accompany the release of toxins. Your body is a wonderful creation equipped with many tools that aid in proper function. The body's ability to release gas is one of these tools.

Bring your hands to the sides of your body, just above your hipbones. Lift, pinch, and roll the flesh here, kneading up and down the sides of your abdomen. Complete the massage of your abdominal area by gently circling the entire area with clockwise strokes.

Shoulders

The relaxation of the abdominal area opens the rest of your body to massage. Remain in a comfortable seated or lying position and move your hands from your abdomen up to your shoulders, lightly resting your hands on them, then gliding down and off. Repeat this gliding stroke across your shoulders three or four times. Stroke the top and back of your shoulders as though you are throwing away any burdens you may be carrying.

Using one hand on the opposite shoulder, start where your shoulder meets your neck, and knead your shoulder between your fingers and thumbs, or between your fingers and the heel of your palm. As you can see in Figure 23, your fingers work on the back of your shoulder while your thumb or heel of your palm works on the inside.

Grasp the skin and muscle along the line of your shoulder, moving out to the edge. Repeat this at least three times on each shoulder.

Now using both hands, place your fingers on both shoulders to press and stroke off. This movement is the same movement you used to start your shoulder massage, but this time your fingers stroke in a different style. Let your fingers press in to the back of your shoulders first and then pull off. Move up from the broad part of your shoulders to your upper shoulder while you press and pull. "Listen" with your fingers to identify any tight areas. If you find tightness, use a friction stroke with small deep circles and narrow in on the troublesome areas. Circle and press until you feel the tightness loosening. Using the same friction stroke on one shoulder at a time, push with your fingertips down the ridge of your shoulder and onto the top of the back. Press and glide along your shoulder to the top of your arm, feeling the tight areas under your fingertips. Repeat. Then move to your other shoulder and press and stroke off, trying to find any tight areas in that shoulder, too.

Moving Down the Arms

With both hands on either side of your neck, brush lightly down from the curve in your neck to the top of your arms, sealing the work you have just performed. Brush with your hands three or four times. Raise your hands up off your shoulders and repeat these strokes.

Stretch out one arm and rest the opposite hand on the top of your outstretched hand. Breathe and begin. Glide your open top hand up your arm to your shoulder and back to your hand several times. Feel your skin and underlying muscles relax with the gentle stroking as you glide over the entire surface of your arm. Grasp your arm between your fingers and your thumb, your fingers on the top side with your thumb on the bottom side, and rub up your arm using a friction stroke. Your skin will feel hot and tingly as your blood circulates to the surface of your arm. Repeat on your other arm.

Now begin kneading your upper arm, starting at the top of your elbow and working up to the shoulder. Using firm, grasping strokes, knead the muscles in the front of your arm and then knead the muscles on the back of your arm. Knead up to your shoulder. Then glide back down your arm, and knead up again, covering the entire surface of your upper arm. Make sure to work the underside of your upper arm right into your underarm area. Massage your underarm area using small circular strokes and round gliding strokes. Repeat on your other arm, starting with gliding strokes from your hand up to your shoulder.

> ### Be Careful of Upper Arms
>
> Because it has soft skin and many lymph nodes, the underarm area is quite sensitive, requiring you to work very slowly and gently. The upper inner arm along the length of the bone must be worked firmly but also gently because this area contains many nerve passageways.

Now work your forearm using the thumb and index finger of your opposite hand, lifting and pinching the skin from your wrist to your elbow, covering your entire forearm. Move from your wrist up to your elbow in a straight line, then glide down to your wrist and work up again in another line. Do this stroke over your entire forearm. Repeat the up-and-down kneading, but this time use all your fingers (not just your index finger) in a grasping and kneading motion, as demonstrated in Figure 24. Your forearm will feel energized.

Make sure you work all around your elbow with kneading and circling strokes. The muscles and tendons in this area are often tight from repetitive motion. Working in the elbow area relieves congestion and stress not only at the elbow but in the entire arm. Move to your other arm and massage in the same way, starting with the lifting and pressing strokes at your wrist.

Massaging Your Hands

Wring your hands together, consciously feeling every part of your hands. Clap your hands together until they tingle. Tap your fingertips and thumbs at least ten times, then press and hold to the count of ten. Extend your arms, turn them slightly so the backs of your hands meet, and then clap. Wring one wrist and then the other at least five times each.

Next, press your index finger into the web between the thumb and index finger of your opposite hand, and hold the other side of the web with your thumb. Using a slight rolling motion press along from the bottom of the web up to the top, holding your hands in the position shown in Figure 25. Repeat on the other hand.

Finally, knead your closed fist into your open palm; then use your fingers to press and circle over your entire open palm. Switch hands and repeat these strokes. Finish by gliding off both palms with soft stroking movements, letting each hand stroke the other as if you are wiping off your hands.

Transitioning to Your Lower Body: Massaging Your Hips

Standing with both hands on your hips, circle in a gliding effleurage movement, warming up the area. With your fingertips on both hips make small deep circles along the hips and buttocks. Cover the entire area and repeat. Now, using your fingers and thumbs lift, pinch, and roll over your hips and buttocks, paying attention to any painful or tight areas. Focus on those areas with your finger pads, pressing and circling each point, then holding for a count of three. Move to each spot at least twice. After this movement, knead again with your fingers and thumbs over the entire hip and buttock area. To finish, circle and glide over the hips and buttocks, covering the area completely.

On to Your Legs!

The hips attach to the legs and provide support for them; the thighbones, shinbones, and ultimately the feet carry the weight of the body. The feet support and balance the body when you walk or stand. It is obvious that these areas get quite a workout and can carry as much, if not more, tension than your arms, shoulders, hands, and abdomen.

Upper Leg: Your Thigh

Sit now as you glide both your hands along one thigh from your hip to your knee and back up again in long circular motions over the front, sides, and back. Next, grasp the flesh and knead up and down your entire thigh, from hip to knee, in an imaginary line along the front, back, and sides. Again, feel for areas of sensitivity, and work deeper in tight areas while using less pressure in areas that are too painful. Repeat on your other thigh.

Sensitive Spots on the Legs

Use caution in the upper thigh and groin area, where the front part of the leg touches the torso. This area is a major pathway for veins and arteries. Too much pressure can cut off circulation. Behind the knee is another area sensitive to pressure, so massage there lightly.

With one hand on the outer thigh of each leg, follow the bones down the sides using circular pressure strokes. When you reach the outer edge of your knees, circle around the tops of the kneecaps and work up your inner thighs. At the top of your thighs, circle and press down the center of your thighs to your knees again. Circle along the tops of your knees to the outside of your thighs; then circle and press up the bones to your hips where you press and hold for a count of three. Repeat this pattern three times.

Massaging one leg at a time, move your hand to the back of your thigh (use the hand on the same side as the thigh you are working). Working from just under your buttock, circle and press down the back of your thigh to the soft tissue behind your knee. Gently stroke the area behind your knee, but do not circle or press. Work back up your thigh, continuing to circle and press imaginary vertical lines from your buttock to the back of your knee, up and down the back of your thigh, until you reach the inner side of your thigh.

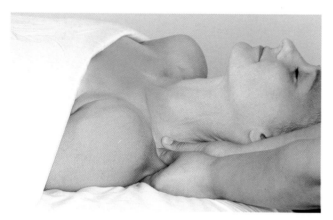

▲ **Figure 1:** Deep muscle kneading. *(Chapter 5)*

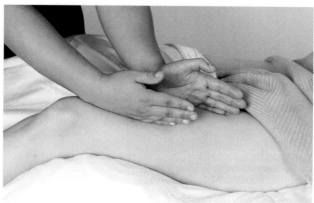

▲ **Figure 2:** Chopping technique. *(Chapter 5)*

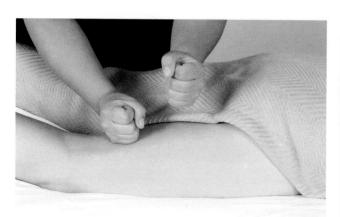

▲ **Figure 3:** Hacking the hamstring muscles.
(Chapter 5)

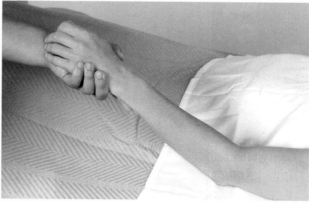

▲ **Figure 4:** Gently hold the wrist to stretch the arm.
(Chapter 5)

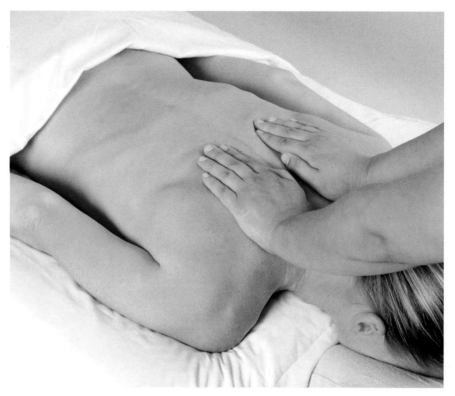

▲ **Figure 5:** Long, gliding stroke on the entire back. *(Chapter 6)*

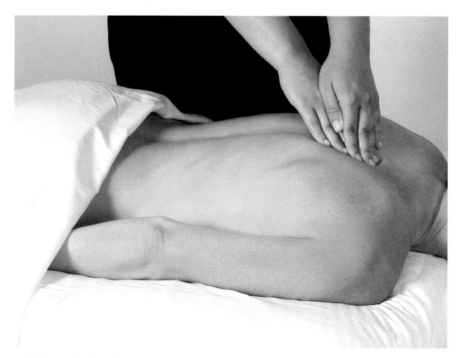

▲ **Figure 6:** Circular stroke to erector muscles along sides of spine.
(Chapter 6)

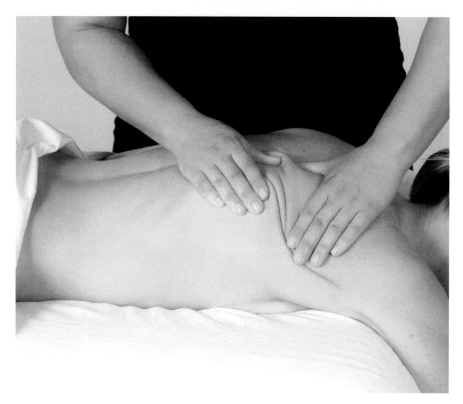

▲ **Figure 7:** Kneading the side of the back. *(Chapter 6)*

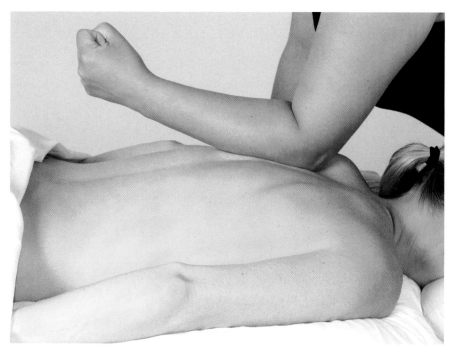

▲ **Figure 8:** Forearm sweeping for mid- and upper back. *(Chapter 6)*

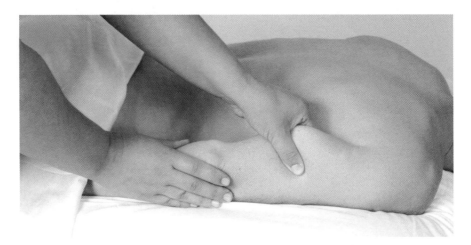

▲ **Figure 9:** Kneading stroke on the back of the upper arm. *(Chapter 6)*

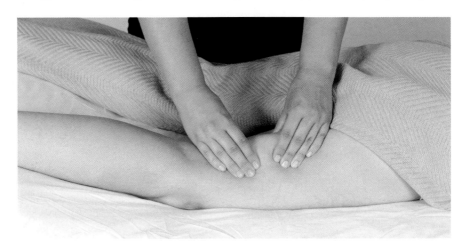

▲ **Figure 10:** Kneading stroke down the back of the leg. *(Chapter 6)*

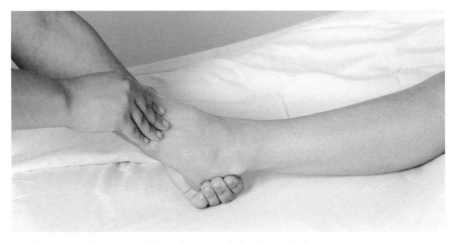

▲ **Figure 11:** Finger stroking the top of the foot. *(Chapter 7)*

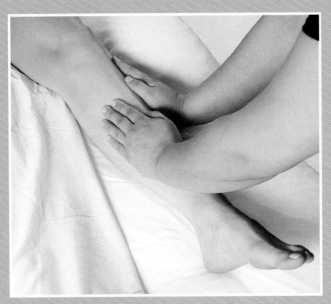

▲ **Figure 12:** Long, gliding strokes from the ankle to the hip. *(Chapter 7)*

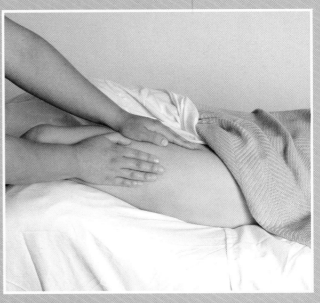

▲ **Figure 13:** Circular kneading up the front of the leg. *(Chapter 7)*

◀ **Figure 14:** Lift and knead the flesh of the thigh. *(Chapter 7)*

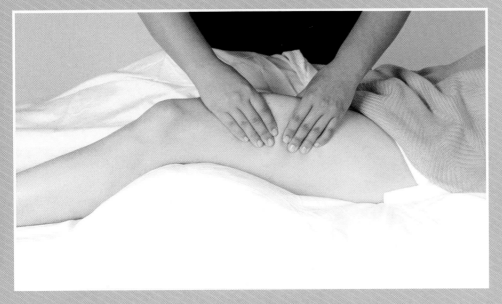

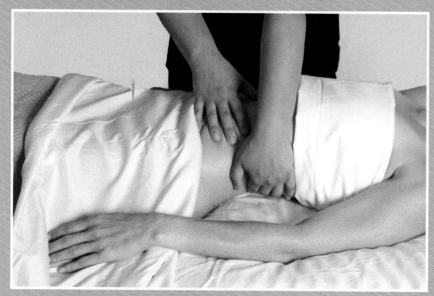

◄ **Figure 15:** Gliding strokes across the abdomen. *(Chapter 7)*

◄ **Figure 16:** Effleurage up the arm. *(Chapter 7)*

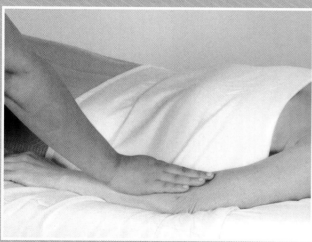

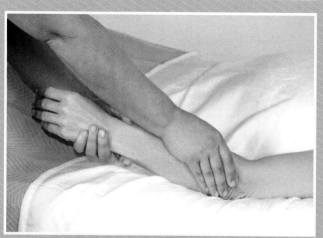

▲ **Figure 17:** Circle on the elbow. *(Chapter 7)*

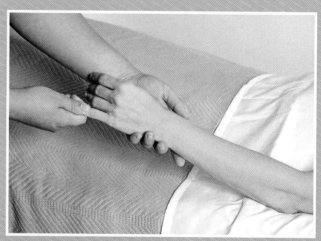

▲ **Figure 18:** Press thumb down fingers. *(Chapter 7)*

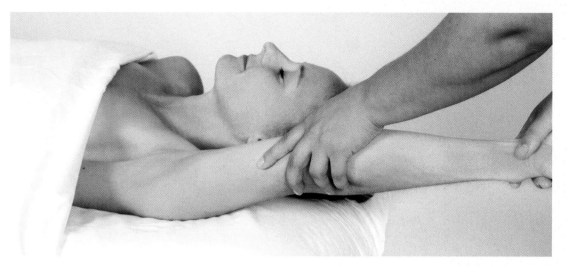

▲ **Figure 19:** Circle the arm at the head. *(Chapter 7)*

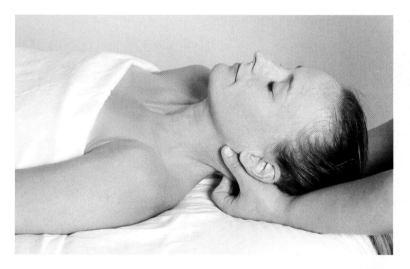

◀ **Figure 20:** The head rests in your hands. *(Chapter 7)*

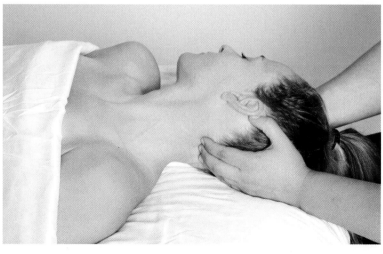

◀ **Figure 21:** Press fingers in at the occipital ridge. *(Chapter 7)*

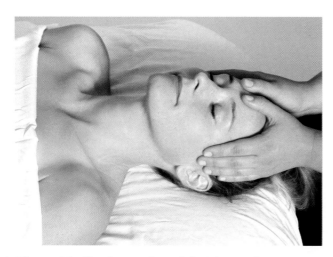

▲ **Figure 22:** Circular motion of thumbs on the forehead. *(Chapter 7)*

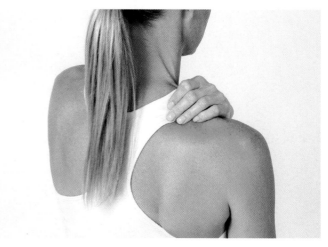

▲ **Figure 23:** Self-massage kneading stroke on shoulder. *(Chapter 10)*

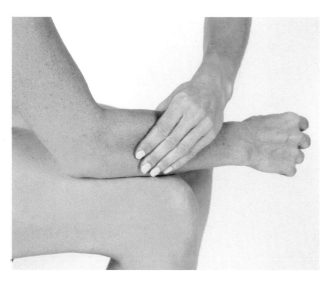

▲ **Figure 24:** Kneading stroke on the forearm. *(Chapter 10)*

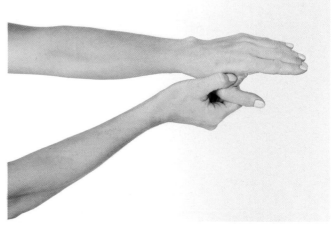

▲ **Figure 25:** Rolling stroke in the web of the thumb. *(Chapter 10)*

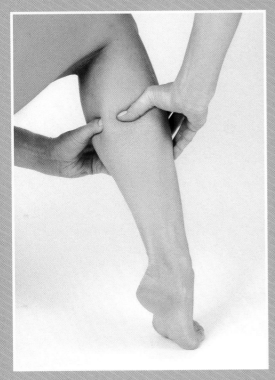

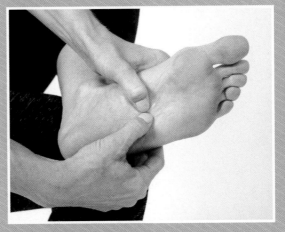

▲ **Figure 26:** Kneading stroke of the calf. *(Chapter 10)*

▲ **Figure 27:** Circular kneading of the sole. *(Chapter 10)*

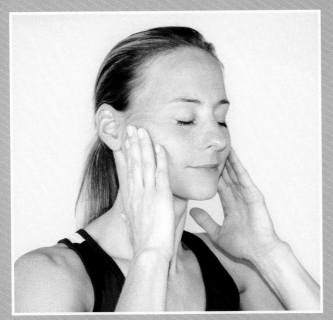

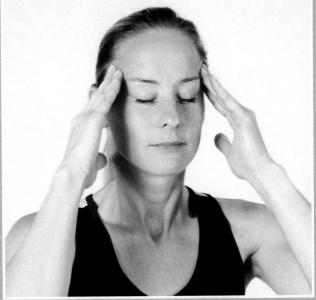

▲ **Figure 28:** Kneading stroke on the cheeks. *(Chapter 10)*

▲ **Figure 29:** Spiral strokes on the head. *(Chapter 10)*

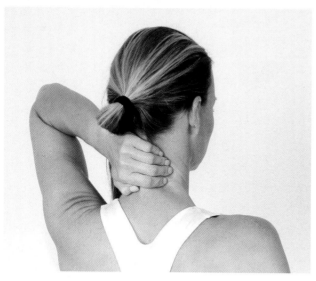

▲ **Figure 30:** Squeezing stroke on the back of your neck. *(Chapter 10)*

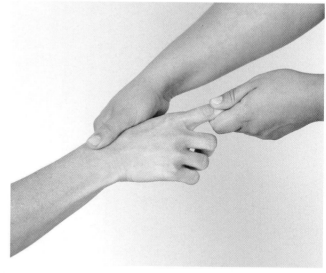

▲ **Figure 31:** Thumb walk down the finger. *(Chapter 11)*

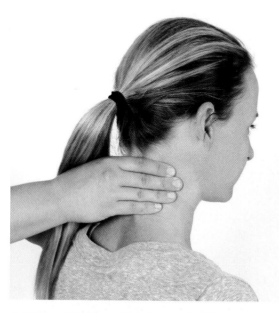

▲ **Figure 32:** Kneading the neck. *(Chapter 11)*

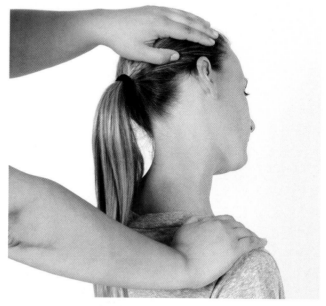

▲ **Figure 33:** Carefully stretch the neck. *(Chapter 11)*

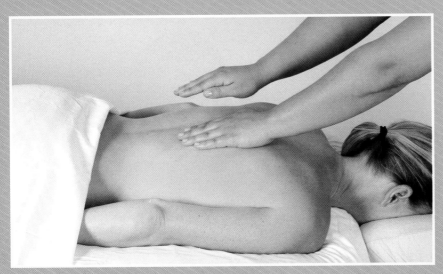

Figure 34: Rest your hands with flat palms. *(Chapter 14)*

Figure 35: Friction of the calf muscle. *(Chapter 14)*

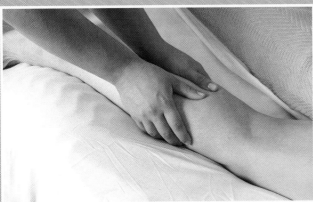

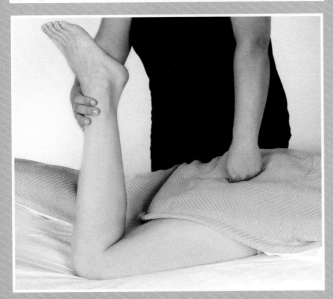

Figure 36: Knead the buttocks. *(Chapter 14)*

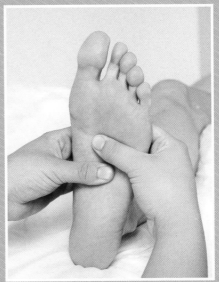

Figure 37: Wringing the foot. *(Chapter 14)*

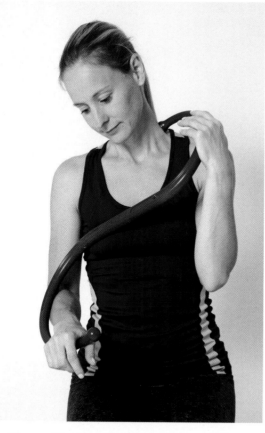

▲ **Figure 38:** Using the Backnobber on the upper trapezius. *(Chapter 17)*

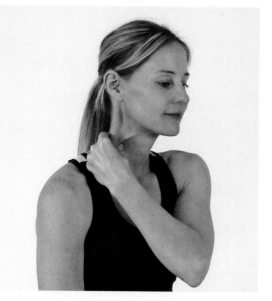

▲ **Figure 39:** Using the pincer technique on the sternocleidomastoid muscle. *(Chapter 17)*

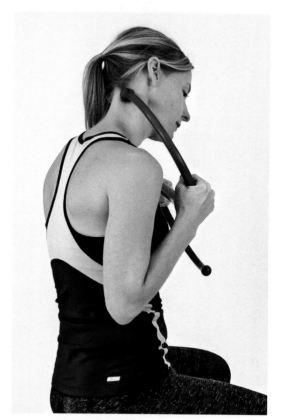

▶ **Figure 40:** Using the Backnobber on suboccipitals. *(Chapter 17)*

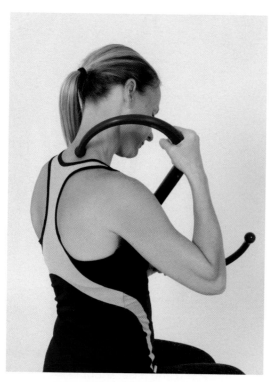

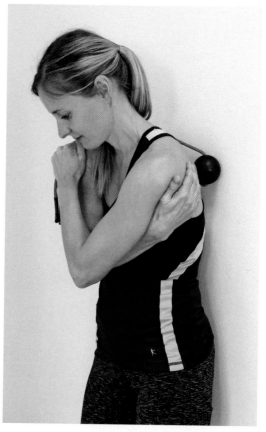

▲ **Figure 41:** Using the Backnobber just next to the upper shoulder blade area. *(Chapter 17)*

▲ **Figure 42:** Using a Tiger Ball on the shoulder blade. *(Chapter 17)*

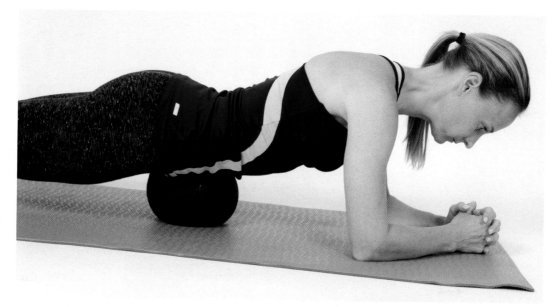

▲ **Figure 43:** Using a FitBall on the abdomen *(advanced)*. *(Chapter 17)*

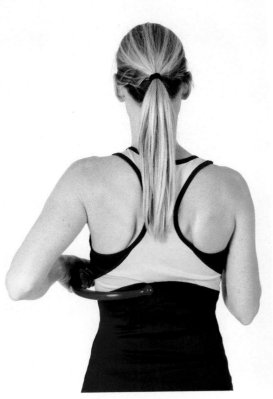

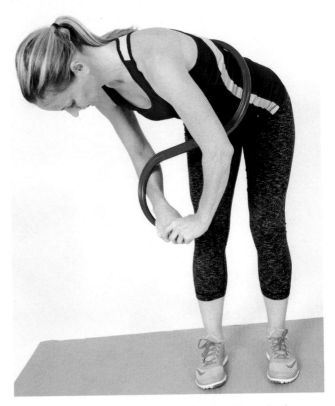

▲ **Figure 44:** Using a Backnobber on the spinal erector muscles. (*Chapter 17*)

▲ **Figure 45:** Using a Backnobber on the spinal erector muscles while bending. (*Chapter 17*)

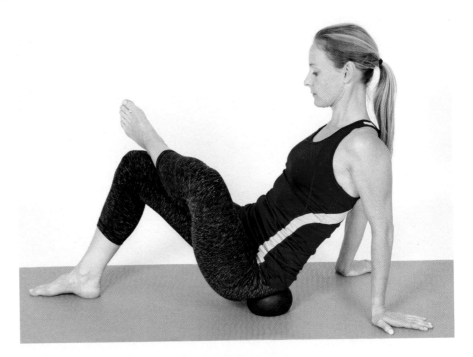

▶**Figure 46:** Using a FitBall on the glutes. (*Chapter 17*)

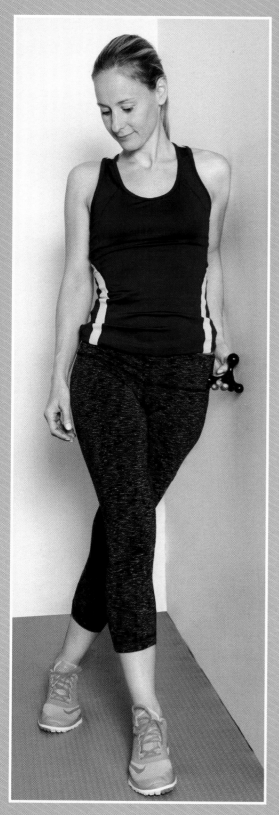

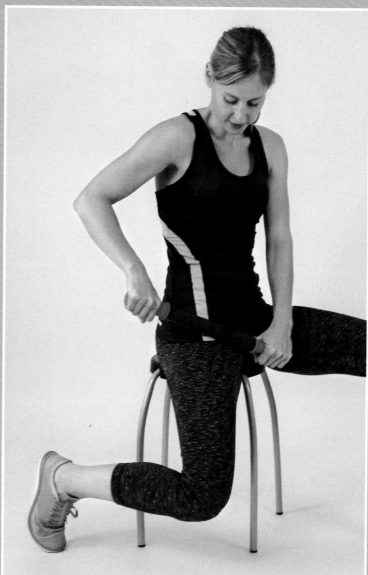

Figure 47: Using a Jacknobber on the hip.
(*Chapter 17*)

Figure 48: Using a Tiger Tail on the thigh.
(*Chapter 17*)

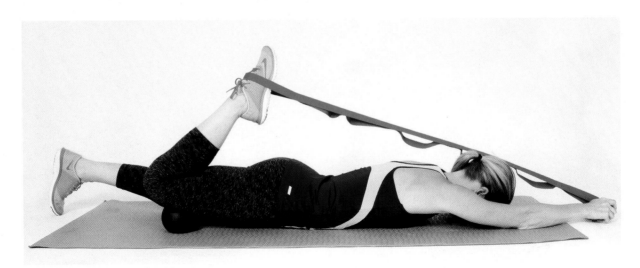

▲ **Figure 49:** Using a strap and FitBall to press on quads. *(Chapter 17)*

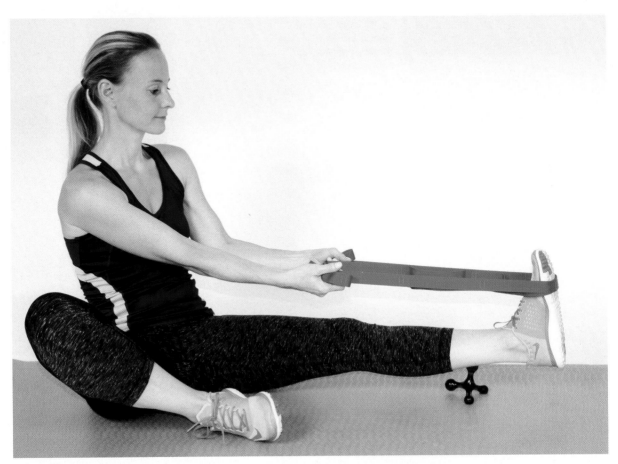

▲ **Figure 50:** Using a Jacknobber on your calf while stretching. *(Chapter 17)*

Using your other hand, press and knead the same thigh in small horizontal lines back and forth across the inner side of your thigh, up to the outer side of your buttock. Then glide over the entire thigh front to back, using deep pressure for two complete gliding strokes. Begin to change the pressure on the third stroke and glide lightly over your upper thigh a few more times for closure. Repeat on the other thigh.

Lower Leg: Your Calf and Shin

To work your calf, either sit and bend forward at your waist or stand and rest your foot on a stool. Using both hands glide over your calf first. Then use both hands to knead the back of your calf from the ankle to the knee, as shown in Figure 26.

As you focus on the center of the calf you may actually feel the two separate parts of the muscle that lie directly under the skin. Use your fingers to press and knead along the centerline in the back of your calf.

What Are Shin Splints?

Shin splints, which is the common name for inflammation of the area where the shin muscle attaches to the shinbone in the front of the lower leg, can cause pain. This can occur as a result of repetitive motion, chronic dehydration, or trigger points in the shin muscle. Overexercising, running, walking up and down hills, or treadmill work may all produce this condition.

Using the pads of your fingers, press and circle down the front of your leg on each side of your shinbone. When you reach the ankle, glide back to the top of your shin and repeat the circles.

Using both hands, press and glide deeply from your ankle up to your knee using your fingers. Press deeply over the entire front and sides of your lower leg, avoiding any pressure on the bone. Lastly, with both hands use your fingers to press deeply with horizontal lines from the ankle to the knee.

Switch legs and work the same routine on your other leg, starting with the gliding stroke over your calf, and kneading the back of your calf from your ankle to your knee.

Your Feet

You will massage the tops, sides, and bottoms of both your feet. Work one foot at a time in a sitting position with your foot crossed over your other leg. Start by pressing and kneading the sole of your foot with a wringing technique, using both hands. Use your thumbs to apply circular friction on the sole, as shown in Figure 27.

With one hand, press your fingers along the sole of your foot in imaginary lines from your heel to your toes. Press your fingers in, slowly moving up your foot. The arch of your foot may be sensitive so apply less pressure there.

Now, using both hands again, circle with your fingers around your ankle, pressing gently and firmly. Work around your entire ankle to the very back of your heel, which is a very sensitive region known as the Achilles' heel; apply firm but gentle pressure there. Smooth the ankle area with circular gliding strokes that evolve into light feathering with just the tips of your fingers touching your ankle.

Next, grasp all your toes with one hand and gently squeeze them and release, applying slight pressure with the heel of your palm. As you stroke along each toe from the bottom to the tip of the nail, one toe at a time, pay attention to the pressure—it should be firm yet gentle. Work the top and bottom of each toe. Grasp all your toes again and gently squeeze. Lastly, stroke gently over the top and bottom of your foot in soft, feathering strokes. Move to your other foot and repeat, starting with pressing and kneading the sole.

Lower Back

This area includes the region below your rib cage to the back of your buttocks. Place both hands behind you, resting your hands between your ribs and your waist. This marks the kidney area. Move your hands down to your tailbone and begin to glide from the center of your body out to the side. Glide in and out as far as you comfortably can as you move up your lower back. Glide down and circle up, three times. Rest your hands at your waistline and knead in to either side of the spine.

Lift, pinch, and press along your waistline, moving down your back to your tailbone. Knead alongside your tailbone, moving out toward the upper curve of your hip. Knead back in and over the entire buttock area. Using an effleurage stroke, gently move up your lower back from your buttocks to the bottom of your rib cage.

Work from your rib cage to the side of your body, kneading as you go. Continue to knead from your spine out to the side to just below the waistline. Knead back and forth along this area at least three times. Use gentle gliding circles to complete your lower back.

> **Avoid the Spine!**
>
> Remember, do not work directly on the spine. The vertebrae (the bones of the spine) house the spinal cord from which all nerves emanate. Never press on this area. These small bones guard the operating system of the body. Massage providers do not adjust bones, chiropractors do.

Face, Head, and Neck

The tension of your daily life is often held in your head and neck, and it shows on your face. By massaging yourself in these areas, you can release the built-up tension and relax your muscles, encouraging yourself to be restful. Massage in general, and working these areas in particular, helps you to slow down and be in the present moment.

To begin, place both your open hands gently on your face as you inhale and exhale. Let your hands rest here through three deep breaths. Circle your hands up and out over either side of your face, using your nose as the dividing line. Glide your entire palms and your fingers smoothly over your skin as you inhale on the up stroke and exhale on the circle out and down stroke. Then use both your hands to glide up your neck from your chest, one hand following the other in long, smooth strokes off the chin.

Now place both hands on the sides of your face, kneading with your fingers from your jaw to your cheeks. As shown in Figure 28, your hands should be pointing up toward your ears as your fingers knead your cheeks.

Continue to knead in small circles over your entire jaw and cheek area. You are releasing any tightness in your jaw as well as stimulating your gums.

Use the same circular kneading with your fingertips from the sides of your nose out to your ears and back again. Feel your sinuses begin to open as the muscles in this area loosen. Using gentle pressure, circle with your fingers from your eyes onto your forehead, making spiral patterns in lines running from your eyebrows out to the sides of your head. Refer to Figure 29 for the position of your fingers.

Using all your fingers, move onto your scalp, circling with small tight strokes up from your forehead. Continue to use the small circle strokes as you work over your entire head, ending up at the bony ridge on either side of your neck at the base of your skull. Place your fingers into the notches on both sides of your neck, and make small circular movements.

Alternate your hands as you hold and squeeze gently on the back of your neck. Check your hand position by referring to Figure 30.

Feel the tightness releasing from your neck. Now place your fingertips back into the notches at the base of your skull, and press in and hold as you count to five. Slowly ease your fingers away as you glide down the back of your neck to your shoulders in sweeping strokes. Massage over your entire scalp and back of your neck again with small circular strokes, ending with the sweeping strokes off your shoulders.

Close with Chakras

The ancient Sanskrit word for wheel is chakra. Chakras are wheels, or circles, of energy that continuously spin in a gentle clockwise fashion, connecting to prominent areas of our bodies. The gentle massage you just gave yourself has affected your entire physical body, and at the same time has affected your chakras, balancing your emotions and your spiritual self. The loving, kind touch you have experienced resounds throughout your entire being. (For a thorough review of chakras, visit ChakraEnergy.com at *www.chakraenergy.com/seven.html*.)

At this moment, you are whole. Your intention to treat yourself with loving kindness has allowed you to release tension and experience a time of simple joy. You are a vital, loving person who has created a healing space within and without. Lie down comfortably if you are able, because this will allow you to totally experience this place you have created. Try to allow yourself to experience the full benefit of your massage.

Lying flat, close your eyes and breathe deeply. Rest your arms at your sides, palms up. Feel your breath cleansing and healing with every inhale and exhale. Imagine your cleansing breath flowing through your body, pushing any toxins out through the palms of your hands and the soles of your feet. Imagine now a strong healing heat flowing through your hands.

Place one hand flat on your pelvic region and the other hand just above it but below your bellybutton. Rest your hands gently, feeling the heat flow from your palms into your body. Empty your mind of busy thoughts and breathe. Think of a soft glowing red light flowing through your bottom hand. Feel its warmth. Through your top hand, imagine an orange light gently flowing into your body. Relax.

The Power of Your Breath

Breathing from the abdomen can create a deep sense of relaxation. As you inhale, life-giving air flows into the lungs. The lungs send oxygen into the blood and take carbon dioxide out. As you exhale, the lungs push out the carbon dioxide and the cycle continues.

Move your bottom hand up above your bellybutton and rest it palm down. Bring your other hand up into the center of your breastbone and place it gently there, palm down. Feel your body under your hands. Concentrate on the heat flowing between your hands and your body. Imagine a yellow light flowing out of the hand on your belly down into your stomach and beyond, spreading warm golden light. From the hand resting on your chest, imagine a brilliant green light radiating into your heart.

Take the hand from your stomach and rest it gently on your throat. Move the hand from your breastbone and rest it on your forehead. Now sense the energy flowing from your hands as the warmth increases. Imagine a sky-blue light flowing into your body from the hand resting on your throat. Imagine a deep indigo-blue light flowing between your eyes from the hand resting on your forehead. Feel these lights as they send soft and nurturing warmth. You are very relaxed yet vibrantly energized.

Now let both your hands rest for a moment on the top of your head. Imagine a deep violet light flowing from your hands down through your entire body. As the violet light moves into every part of you, rest your arms at your sides, palms up. Feel the peace that is flowing through your body. Enjoy it, embrace it, and remember it.

You have touched and awakened the healer within. Celebrate this part of yourself often. Remember to breathe and stretch and to love yourself always. Enjoy the wonderfulness that is you with yourself and with others.

Chapter 11
Chair Massage

The Evolution of Chair Massage

Chair massage has allowed the field of touch to enter into the office, the airport, sports events, concerts, malls, and the offices of medical professionals. You will find chair-massage therapists volunteering their services during medical disasters and emergencies. The relaxation and pain relief receivers experience from a ten- to twenty-minute seated massage promotes a sense of well-being and productivity that typically surpasses all expectations.

Early massage therapists in the United States were trained in many modalities including shiatsu, amma, and tui na. These are bodywork techniques practiced by Eastern cultures since ancient times. These therapies, although not technically massage, were required subjects for practitioners of massage, and all could be performed, at least in part, with the recipient in a seated position. Massage therapists developed new techniques based on this seated approach, and some early therapists brought these techniques into the workplace, offering a professional, seated massage to employees in large companies.

Massage schools began to recognize the variety of uses that seated massage could provide and developed curricula to service that need. In the late 1970s, a massage professional demonstrated her seated technique to attendees at a national massage conference, sparking further interest in this method. As a result, training programs in massage began to reflect the variety of populations served by massage, including seated massage, and eventually established a protocol for seated massage, which allows the service to be offered to everyone, regardless of physical restrictions.

> ### Ancient Chair Massages
>
> Seated massage has origins that can be traced to ancient China. More than 3,000 years ago, the Chinese discovered points that trigger healing responses when touched. This discovery spread throughout the Eastern world, influencing healing work in Japan and India as well. Many of these traditional styles included a form of seated massage as part of the treatment.

Educators, parents, and massage therapists, realizing the value of seated massage, began to look for and develop programs offering this technique. Populations of children and adults with disabilities began to receive this style of massage. Employees in large corporations were encouraged to take advantage of corporate-sponsored chair massages. The practice of easing our tired backs by rubbing them on a chair eventually caught on.

Chair Massage Today

A massage therapist named David Palmer worked to promote chair massage during the early 1980s. At first Palmer's group had a minimal amount of success promoting his chair-massage service to the business world. However, in 1984 Palmer acquired Apple Inc. as a client, and the chair-massage practitioners found their niche. Today, this accessible method of massage is relaxing thousands of people daily, not only in the workplace but also in countless other arenas.

Unlike traditional massage, which is generally private, chair massage is very visible. This allows bystanders to observe what takes place and know what to expect if they decide to try it. It has taken the mystery and fear out of bodywork, plus it is easy to receive and it is inexpensive. What could possibly be scary about sitting in a chair with all your clothes on in a public place getting a back rub? And what could be more convenient? For many, chair massage is their introduction into the healing world of skilled, compassionate touch.

In the Office or on the Road

Chair massage offers a time-saving and inexpensive approach to stress relief. This approach to massage offers a welcome break in the middle of a busy day, without caffeine or nicotine! Recipients of chair massage do not have to worry about being undressed, either. Although skilled, compassionate touch is wonderful, many people feel uncomfortable undressed or partially undressed, even draped with a cover. Chair massage offers a healthy alternative and an acceptable introduction into the remarkable world of massage.

Corporate Massage

The introduction of chair massage into the world of fast pace, fast money, and fast demands has provided a remarkable doorway for change within the corporate setting.

The work ethic of most Americans is work until you drop, providing your company with the best output you can produce. The integrity of most workers is impeccable and deserves to be rewarded, as most owners of companies realize.

Chair massage provides a healthy break from the stress of the workplace. Fortunately, many companies understand the benefits of chair massage and the resulting increase in overall productivity. The brief time an employee spends receiving a chair massage reaps incredible rewards for both the employee and the company.

> **Sitting Can Create Repetitive Muscle Strain!**
> Any part of the body that repeats the same motion over a period of time may develop trigger points and strain in the muscles. This painful state limits mobility and restricts the use of the area until the muscle strain is rehabilitated. Muscles that stay in one position for an extended period of time can also develop trigger points and tension. Chair massage helps to prevent these conditions.

On-site chair massage from a licensed professional provides a restful yet invigorating release of tension, creating an atmosphere of camaraderie that promotes resourcefulness and productivity. Ask your human resources department if your company offers such a perk.

Travel Massage

Massage on the road is made easy with a seated routine. Anything that can be turned into a seat can be used as a tool for massage. Those who travel either for business or pleasure can give each other seated massage using a stool, a portable camping chair, or a blanket on the ground. Anyone can massage your shoulders and neck, releasing tension and stored energy while freeing stiff muscles and helping loosen tight muscles that may cause pain.

Other Environments

The opportunities available to provide chair massage are endless:

- Conventions and meeting centers are great places to offer chair massage.
- Charity events love to offer chair massage as a fundraising gift.
- Hospitals use chair massage for their staff, providing a calm and quiet space for the healers to be healed.
- Truck drivers and construction workers receive tremendous benefits from chair massage, as do the operators of buses and trains.
- Waitstaff, dishwashers, cooks, and bartenders are on their feet all day, and a chair massage can provide them much needed healing.

Chair Massage Is Inexpensive

Chair massage has no added expense, because you do not have to buy oils or use linens to drape. You can buy a dedicated massage chair if you wish, but it is not necessary. Remember to stretch after you give the massage to release any tension you may have created doing the work.

Advantages of Chair Massage

Massage of any type is fantastic, but there are many people who do not want to take off their clothes, never mind the part about lying on a table with their faces down, waiting for someone they don't know to rub them with oil. Even if the person giving the massage is a dear friend, she just might not like to get undressed for a massage. Chair-massage recipients are fully clothed and sit in a chair while the giver targets areas of tension without using oil. The giver of the massage either brings a chair made for chair massage or improvises with whatever chair is available. Regardless, no one has to lie down on a table. Because the recipient is fully clothed and in a less vulnerable position than in traditional massage, this technique may even help eliminate someone's fear and worry of being touched.

Others can't seem to justify taking an hour solely for themselves. Chair massage, although highly effective, is brief, perhaps fifteen to twenty minutes, and can be done on a coffee break. Chair massage is usually conducted out in the open, which reinforces the feeling of safety in those who are somewhat timid. Massage given in the workplace lowers stress and, as a result, the number of stress-related illnesses. It also promotes a sense of well-being, and ultimately helps raise productivity.

Techniques for Chair Massage

The strokes used in chair massage are a combination of Eastern acupressure and Swedish massage techniques. You will use a combination of acupressure, trigger point pressure release, compression, friction, stretching, petrissage, effleurage, tapping, and feather strokes, all applied through the clothes without oil. Your goal is to release the tension that can sit in the back, shoulders, neck, hands, and arms. You will also try to release trigger points and relieve muscle stress and congestion. Overall, of course, you will be providing relaxation.

Using Acupressure and Trigger Point Compression

Acupressure, or any type of held compression, is the application of steady pressure to an affected area for the purpose of stretching the muscle and releasing congested fluid buildup from the tissues. The pressure is applied and held on a spot by your finger, thumb, elbow, or forearm, or sometimes all your fingers. Holding on a trigger point helps to break up muscle spasms. This static technique works in conjunction with other techniques like friction and kneading petrissage.

Compression can also be applied with the heels of your hands or elbow in a steady, even, press-and-hold technique. Stabilize yourself at the part of the body being massaged, and press down firmly. Hold for a moment, coordinate your release with the receiver's exhale if you can, and release. Then press again into another nearby area, moving in small increments over the area being worked.

Using Friction

Friction is the movement of skin over muscle, and can be applied in a variety of styles. One way is to place both your hands on the area, palms down, and move back and forth in a sliding movement over the region. This quickly warms up the muscles underneath. Use this movement along either side of the spine, on the broad area of the back, along the shoulders, or up the arms.

Another way to apply friction is more of an isolating move. Rather than gliding across the skin, press your fingers into the muscles, hold, and push the skin over the muscles as you move your fingers. By pressing you are able to reach in deeper. As you become more familiar with this movement, you can actually feel the muscle underneath. This type of friction works well with acupressure, because it allows you to focus on specific pressure points.

Using Stretching

There are three ways to use stretching in chair massage:

1. One way is an **active assisted stretch**, which means you help your receiver stretch a tiny bit more. For example, gently pull the receiver's arm as she stretches to open up the shoulder a little more.
2. Another is an **active resisted stretch**, which means your receiver resists the stretch as you gently pull.
3. The last one is the **passive stretch**, which means you do all the stretching while the person being worked on lets it happen. Be careful; do not push or pull aggressively. The passive stretch should be a smooth, gentle stretch that helps the muscle loosen. Pull gently, stop, and check with the receiver to see if the stretch is within his or her comfort range.

> ### Stretching Safety
>
> Be careful when you apply any stretching technique—move only as far as the joint will allow. The range of motion for any joint is how far it will stretch in any direction without causing discomfort. Do not move past that limit or you will injure the receiver.

Using Petrissage

Petrissage is the kneading, rolling, twisting, squeezing, lifting, and pinching technique that gets in and breaks up the congestion. Petrissage can be applied in a number of ways. One style is deep kneading with the hands, which begins by lifting the flesh up into the palms and squeezing, using your fingers to push the skin. Lift, roll, and squeeze, grasping the flesh as you move along the area. As one hand pushes the flesh in, the other hand does the squeezing.

Another common petrissage technique is pinching with your thumb and fingers. Pick up the skin between your thumb and fingers, and roll along as your thumb pushes more flesh into your fingers that are pinching in a constant rock-and-roll motion. Although it is important to move your body as you apply any massage stroke, kneading in particular feels better to the receiver when it is combined with your body movement.

Using Effleurage and Feather Touch

Effleurage is used in chair massage to begin and end the session, as well as to assess the underlying tension. How firmly you glide depends on the "eyes" in your hands as they feel and find where to glide deeper and where to stroke lightly. To glide more deeply, mold your hands to the body as you press along the surface in a smooth rhythmic motion. To glide with a soft, feather touch gently brush your fingertips or palms along the region to calm the nerves. Effleurage may be used over most parts of the body, though it is an especially valuable technique for performing chair massage because your hands can glide easily over clothing.

Using Tapotement

Tapotement in the form of tapping is useful in chair massage for the neck, head, and shoulders. Use your fingers to tap with either light or heavy pressure in these areas—either one feels good. Hacking (karate chops) works wonders on a tight back. Remember to keep your wrists loose and your hands limp, letting the sides of your hands and fingers do the work. You can also apply tapping with a loose fist, easily tapping over a broad surface. Cupping with your hands and tapping over the entire back provides added stimulation. Tapping is best applied by establishing a rhythm and moving over the area in time with the steady beat you have chosen.

A Chair-Massage Routine

Remember, you do not have to buy a formal massage chair to give someone a chair massage. Simply turn a straight-back chair around and place a pillow on the back of the chair for the receiver to rest his or her head. You could also use a stool or chair in front of a table or desk. Place the receiver on the stool with his or her head and arms resting on a pillow (or folded towel) on the table or desktop. Drummer or doctors' stools are great because you can adjust the height to fit the person.

Begin the chair massage by leaning in toward the upper back and pressing your hands down on the shoulders in greeting. Press down with your palms and glide along the shoulder line out to the tops of the arms. Repeat this gliding stroke pressing down and away, relaxing the neck and shoulders. With both hands working together, lift and squeeze the flesh from the neck across the shoulders in a kneading stroke.

Return to the top of the neck, placing the first two fingers of each hand into the notch on either side of the spine at the base of the skull. Press down alongside the spine, using steady, firm acupressure strokes, all the way to the lower back. Do not press on the spine; make sure you are on either side at the edge of the vertebrae.

Return to the shoulders again and place one palm flat on the shoulder blade while you press down along the opposite side of the spine with two fingers. Repeat this technique on the other side, and remember to move your body as you work.

Lean in toward the receiver as you hold one shoulder with your forearm while you circle with friction over the other side of the back, working from the recipient's shoulders to the hips. Holding the opposite shoulder allows you to stabilize muscle and stretch the skin on the other side. Switch to the other side and repeat.

The Arms

Stand in front of the chair as you hold the recipient's arm with both hands. Rest the arm on your forearm as you glide over the entire arm with your other hand, turning it so you can touch all parts. Using both your hands, squeeze up and down the arm, stimulating the muscles. Next, use one hand to knead along the muscles of the upper arm, again supporting the arm with your other hand. One hand does the work while the other supports the arm.

Now hold the arm under the elbow and under the wrist, and stretch. Remember to stop before you feel resistance. Then gently shake the arm, and feel the muscles relax. While you are holding the receiver's hand, press down the length of each finger and circle around the wrist. Remember not to pull the fingers, but rather support the wrist and slowly walk with your thumb down every finger. Refer to Figure 31 to check your position when working on the hand.

Return the arm gently to the receiver's side and repeat these strokes on the other arm.

Hips and Lower Back

When working on the lower back and hips you may find that kneeling or squatting works best for you. Lightly glide both hands down the recipient's back from the neck to the hips, two or three times. Then press along the side of the spine with your thumbs or fingers, starting below the rib cage and working right to the hipbones. Now move out from the center of the back and press along the buttocks out to the sides of the hips. Continue this pressing move, returning to the center and circling out until you have covered the entire lower back and hips.

Next, use your palms and press into the lower back and all along the buttocks and hips. The heels of the palms will do most of the work with your fingers gliding along. Move each hand away from the center, pressing out.

Keep the Lines of Communication Open

Remember to keep an ongoing check with your receiver. Whenever you move to a new section of the body, ask how the pressure is and how the recipient is feeling overall. When trying something new, go slowly, keeping within the comfort range of the receiver.

For this next movement, work one side of the body and then the other. Again you will need to kneel or squat as you press with your thumbs or fingers along the side of the thigh from the hip to the knee. Press up and down along the thigh from the knee to the hip, working to the center of the thigh. Repeat these acupressure strokes back out to the side of the leg, then feather off. Move to the other leg and follow the same steps.

The Neck and Head

Standing behind the receiver, place both hands on either side of the receiver's neck and then glide down and off the shoulders, using steady, smooth pressure. Follow this by pressing two fingers in at the base of the skull and pressing to the bottom of the neck. Return your fingers to the top of the neck and press down again until you have covered the entire neck. Ask your receiver if the pressure is fine or if you need to ease up a bit.

Next, knead the neck by lifting and squeezing the neck muscles with one hand, pushing the flesh into your palm with your thumbs as you squeeze with your fingers, as shown in Figure 32.

Move down to knead the neck muscles that flow into the back. These hold a tremendous amount of tension. Finally, gently stretch the neck by holding one side at the top of the shoulder and gently guiding the stretch by a slight press to the head, as shown in Figure 33. Stretch the neck to the left side and back to the center, and then over to the right side and back to the center again.

Massage the scalp and hair with both hands using circular friction. The tips of your fingers act as though you are shampooing the head of your receiver. The movement is firm without gliding as your fingers lift from each section and move to the next. Then place your hands firmly on the head and gently knead by pressing in and moving the entire palm as you move gently over the entire scalp. Kneading is a great stroke to relieve slight pressure in the head.

The Finish

Tapping over the entire area you just massaged helps to announce the finish of the session. It also invigorates the receiver. Begin with finger tapping from the receiver's head down to the buttocks and over the arms. Then, with your fists slightly closed, beat a gentle percussion stroke over the receiver's back and shoulders.

Next, cup and slap each shoulder and arm with a steady beat, and follow this stroke onto the thighs. Glide your palms smoothly down both sides of the back; then press both your palms firmly on the shoulders, signaling the end.

Chapter 12
Pregnancy and Massage

Why Prenatal Massage Is So Important

To be pregnant is miraculous; to find relief from the various discomforts that may accompany pregnancy is phenomenal. Massage is a marvelous tool that can be used to assist the expectant mother. Indeed, massage during pregnancy is practiced in most cultures throughout the world. Massage provides relief from the discomforts of pregnancy as well as support through the profound changes experienced by the pregnant woman. Massage is a tool of exchange that can be used by both expectant parents. Kind touch communicates love and acceptance, and provides comfort and intimacy.

Pregnancy places a tremendous amount of pressure on the expectant mom's back, abdomen, shoulders, pelvis, legs, and feet, all of which must adapt to carrying the growing baby within. In addition, physiological changes create adverse stress for the mother-to-be as her arteries, veins, and lymph vessels increase their activity and hormones start pumping through her system.

The onset of pregnancy activates the secretion of the hormone relaxin. This hormone works to make the ligaments in the body looser and the joints more mobile. The joints and ligaments connecting the pelvic bones need to loosen, giving the cervix the ability to dilate and the pelvis the ability to stretch during the birth process. Relaxin is not discriminatory, therefore *all* the joints and ligaments in the body loosen during pregnancy. This may result in a variety of problems, such as slipped vertebrae, joint and muscle pain, interrupted nerve supply to muscles, or uneven hip joints. In response to the loosening, muscles may tighten to support and stabilize the joints, resulting in muscle spasms.

Benefits of Prenatal Massage

Prenatal massage works to relieve the stressors that pregnancy imposes upon the body by helping the woman take charge of herself, her body, and her experience in pregnancy. The relaxation provided with massage is profound. As you massage someone who is pregnant, you help to lower her elevated heart and breathing rate, creating a serene environment for the mother to be. Prenatal massage is beneficial in many aspects and creates an overall state of well-being. Some of the specific benefits of massage are that it can:

- Stabilize hormone levels.
- Increase overall circulation.
- Increase blood and oxygen supply.
- Stimulate lymphatic movement.
- Control varicose veins.
- Reduce swelling.
- Lower anxiety.
- Improve sleep.
- Relieve pressure from back and shoulders.
- Promote nerve health.

Contraindications

Massage is essential in an uncomplicated pregnancy, but it can be harmful to certain pregnant women under certain circumstances. That is why it is very important for you to be sure any pregnant woman you plan to massage has gotten approval from her medical practitioner that massage is okay for her. There are specific conditions for which massage is not beneficial. Send a pregnant woman to her doctor if she tells you she has any of the following:

- High blood pressure
- Excessive swelling
- Toxemia
- Morning sickness, nausea, or vomiting
- High fever
- Abdominal pain
- Vaginal bleeding
- High risk of miscarriage
- A high-risk pregnancy, such as placental abruption or preterm labor

Avoid Some Massage Techniques

Increased blood volume can make blood flow sluggish for a pregnant woman. This could put a pregnant woman at risk of blood clots in the lower leg. Blood clots most commonly lodge in the calves or inner thigh. Using strong pressure in these areas could dislodge a blood clot, which is very dangerous. Play it safe and use very light, slow strokes on the legs. When using these light stroking techniques on the legs, begin at the feet and move upward toward the heart. As you work, avoid these massage techniques altogether: deep-tissue massage, deep trigger point pressure release, acupressure, shiatsu, cross-fiber friction, and percussive tapping.

If you choose to massage the belly, only use very light pressure. Some massage therapists do not massage the abdomen at all.

Massage During Labor

There are many signs that alert the expectant mother that she is approaching delivery of her child. Many women feel a sense of excitement and a surge of energy. Often this burst of energy is accompanied by behavior associated with an instinct known as nesting. The need to prepare the nest by cleaning the house and making last-minute adjustments to the nursery space are behaviors attributed to this instinct.

The expectant mom may experience deep lower back pain along with aching legs and pressure low in the pelvis. Her breasts may become more enlarged and heavier as the nourishing milk increases in anticipation of the coming birth.

What Is Dilation?

The opening of the cervix is known as dilation. In stage-one labor—the dilation stage—the cervix dilates to 7 cm, signaling the transition to stage two, the birth. Transition is complete when the cervix is dilated to 10 cm.

The Three Stages of Labor

Labor has three stages, each with very clear identifying features. The first stage starts when the cervix becomes thin and begins to open. There are very distinct contractions at this stage that serve to open the cervix wider in preparation for birth. Stage-one contractions can last for several hours, and usually last longer if this is a first baby.

Staying mobile helps with stage-one labor. If the woman in labor can walk, doing so will speed up her labor and help her ride out the contractions more easily. During the early phase of stage-one labor, deep, slow breathing is helpful in dealing with the contractions. As contractions increase in intensity during the transition phase of stage one, breathing speeds up to a rapid panting as the woman works through each contraction.

The stage-two labor is the actual birth. Contractions come two to five minutes apart and the mother actively pushes during this period, bearing down with each contraction. After the baby is born, contractions continue until the placenta, or afterbirth, is expelled.

The contractions following birth are stage-three labor, also known as the placental stage. These final contractions push out the placenta and constrict blood vessels that were torn during the delivery.

Massage in All Stages

Massage can be an important tool in every stage of labor. During the first stage of labor, loving touch through massage helps the laboring woman feel more confident and supported. As she moves into the transition phase, massage helps to reduce anxiety and bring relief from muscle contractions during this heightened time of pain.

> ### Ask First!
> Massage can be a useful tool during labor, but only if the woman in labor wishes to be touched. Always ask before attempting to administer massage to a woman who is in any stage of labor.

The giver of massage during labor provides a welcome oasis of calmness during a time that can feel isolating and out of control. Loving touch comforts and supports, and also creates a safe space. Caring touch helps the laboring woman to focus, giving her control of her body at a moment that seems without center. Massage gives strength and promotes endurance.

The placental stage is a wonderful time to give massage. The uterine contractions are still quite powerful, and you can assist in the delivery of the afterbirth by massaging the mother's belly. Steady rhythmic massage helps the mother expel the placenta so she may cuddle and rest with her baby.

Following Birth

Massage is also helpful during the weeks of recovery following birth. This postpartum period is the time during which the woman's body returns to its normal prepregnancy state. Hormone levels even out and rebalance. As the hormonal balance is re-established, women often experience physical, emotional, and spiritual changes.

Postpartum Blues

Following birth, as the hormones work to regain balance, many women experience fatigue and the blues, which generally surface within ten days of the delivery. Postpartum emotions can surface as extreme highs and lows, mood swings that may seem irrational. Some women may seem irritable and anxious with no patience for anyone other than the baby. Tearfulness is a response to many situations during this period, and at times sadness may surface. Most women overcome the malaise by returning to a routine of proper rest and nutrition along with support from their communities. Massage helps the mother to heal, too.

Some women experience postpartum depression, a far more severe consequence of the hormonal imbalance that wreaks havoc in the new mother's body. This depression is more serious than the "baby blues." The woman suffering from postpartum depression undergoes mood swings, has difficulty concentrating, and may be anxious and irritable yet cannot express these emotions. Women who suffer with this depression feel unable to cope with their new infant; they feel powerless and inadequate. Anyone with these or similar symptoms should seek professional help. The use of compassionate touch through massage is a useful tool for providing additional support during this trying time.

Benefits of Massage after the Birth

A universal truth is that massage heals, and in cultures throughout the world massage is provided before, during, and after birth. After the birth, a new mother can massage her own belly to help with the production of lochia and the release of this discharge. Massage localized to the abdomen helps speed up the healing of the uterus and helps restore the elasticity of the skin. Massage of the lower back relieves tension. Overall, massage relieves muscle aches and pains, and helps the mother regain energy and strength.

> ### Toxin Removal
>
> As the hormones return to balance, any excess hormones will leave the body as waste, resulting in a heavy volume of urine and excess perspiration. This release of toxins is accompanied by the production of lochia, a normal vaginal discharge that follows birthing. This discharge eventually disappears about two weeks after the birth.

Pregnancy Massage Essentials

Massage during all stages of pregnancy helps the expectant mother maintain her health and sustain her energy level. Pregnancy is a joyous time when the body undergoes many changes as it provides protection and support for the baby. The growing child within creates an ever-changing environment for the mother-to-be.

Strokes for Pregnancy

The basic massage techniques you use on a pregnant woman are ones you have already learned, including effleurage, petrissage, tapotement, friction, and feathering. But as indicated previously, do not use these techniques on the foot, lower leg, or thigh! These include basic Swedish massage strokes as well as a few other techniques derived from Eastern bodywork. If you want to review some of these basic massage techniques, see Chapter 5.

Positioning the Receiver

The mother may feel pressure on the abdomen fairly early in the pregnancy, so begin with the mother lying on her back, with a pillow under her knees for support. Some women may need more than one pillow under their knees and legs. A large pillow to elevate the head and upper back may be more comfortable for some women. As the expectant woman moves toward full term, even lying on her back may become problematic. The growing baby within may press on the descending aorta and interfere with blood flow to the placenta. Always defer to the judgment of the woman.

> ### The Aorta and Its Branches
>
> The aorta is the main artery supplying blood throughout the body. There are many branches that stem from the aorta. One of these branches, the descending aorta, is the branch that feeds the chest, the diaphragm, and the abdominal regions of the body. Too much pressure on this part of the body can interfere with the circulation through this artery.

Ultimately the pregnant woman feels best on her side, and the massage will need to be modified accordingly. However, for now, begin with the mother on her back if she is comfortable in that position.

A Simple Head and Neck Routine

Several components of the pregnancy massage routine are easy to perform on yourself, including the face and ear massage. This not only gives you a chance to practice your technique and become aware of how the receiver feels, but you will also experience some relaxation.

The Face

Use natural oil like jojoba oil and warm it in your hands before applying. (Always ask first; some people will prefer cream on the face and others like nothing at all.) Begin by applying gliding strokes up the neck and off the side of the jaw. Use both hands, one on each side of the face. Continue gliding onto the chin and up over the cheekbones. Glide up the forehead and off the head.

Return to the chin, still using both hands, and use light pinching to lift the flesh up along the jaw to behind the cheekbone. Continue to pinch and lift along the entire chin and cheekbone until the area is covered. Use very easy pinching strokes on the upper lip between the lip and the nose. Press with your index fingers on either side of the nose up to the forehead. Pinch along the ridge of the eyebrow from the outside of the face to the bridge of the nose, and then pinch back from the ridge to the edge of the brow.

> ### Be Watchful of Pregnancy Edema
> Massage affects the flow of fluid in the body. You do not want to push blood through a system that is experiencing a chemical or mechanical breakdown. In cases of extreme swelling, called edema, don't massage—you could make the situation worse.

Using all your fingertips, press from the top of the brow to the top of the forehead. Repeat this movement until the entire forehead has been worked. Now move up to the scalp and rub the entire head using a shampoo motion. At the base of the skull use your fingertips to hook under the two notches directly behind the ears. Gently press into the depression and hold with your hands cupping the back of the head.

The Ears

Place your thumbs behind each ear, resting your thumb pads along the back of the ears; rest your index fingers on the sides of the cheeks in front of the ears. Gently stroke the edge of your index fingers along the entire surface of each ear. This will feel very soothing to the receiver. Grasp each earlobe, with your thumbs on back and index fingers pressing from the other side. Hold this position to a count of five.

Continue to work up along the edge of the ears, with your thumbs on the back side and your index fingers on the inner side of each ear. Slightly pinch along the outside ridges of the ears. At the top of the ears, press your thumbs and index fingers together, and hold to a count of five. Bring your thumbs behind the fleshy lobes and rub your index fingers on the outsides of each lobe. Stroke down the entire lobes of both ears for two minutes; this will relax the whole body.

> **Don't Forget the Ears!**
>
> Working on the ears is actually a soothing reflexology technique that fits very well into massage. The reflexology points of the ear relax the spine and back, as well as the internal organs. Stroking the lobe produces overall relaxation.

The Neck

Relax both your hands along the front of the woman's neck, gently stroking from the clavicle bones to the shoulders. Using both your hands gently glide from the base of the neck up to the chin, holding the chin in an easy stretch for the count of three. Carefully turn the head to one side and, using the fingers of both your hands, glide along the side of the neck up to the base of the skull. Repeat along this area using circular stretching strokes.

Turn the head to the other side and repeat the gliding and circling strokes. Move the head back to the center and place both hands under the base of the skull, cradling the head. Using all your fingers press, pull, and circle from the shoulder line up to the back of the skull, gently stretching at the head. Repeat this stroke at least three times. Lastly, stroke under the head with one hand following the other three times, finally letting the head rest.

Massaging the Body

Massage can relax the expectant mother, releasing muscle tightness and helping to reduce tension. Massage increases levels of the "feel-good" hormones serotonin and dopamine. These hormones make us all feel relaxed and more content.

As circulation is improved and relaxation ensues, the flow of blood and accompanying lymph drainage keeps the muscles and connective tissues healthy. Remember to use sufficient oil to keep your strokes smooth and gentle throughout the entire massage.

The Torso

Cover the woman's breasts with a towel or pillowcase, leaving the stomach uncovered, and let the cover drape everything below the stomach. Place the palms of both your hands flat on the chest just below the collarbone and press. This is a comforting compression move that releases built-up tension in the neck and chest muscles. Now move to the right side of the mother, gently placing your hands on her abdomen.

> **Keep Pressure Gentle**
>
> Never press hard on anyone's abdominal area, especially a pregnant woman's. In a pregnant woman, the organs move around as the baby grows, and the growing child is close to the surface of the abdomen. While massage is beneficial for the baby and the mother, any pressure must be gentle. You must abide by the woman's wishes and use only very gentle gliding strokes if she gives you permission.

Move both your hands in a clockwise manner as you gently stroke with soft gliding motions over the entire abdominal area. Circle up to the ribs and down to the top of the pubic bone; circle up and back again. Always use slow, steady, and gentle strokes. You may even feel the baby moving as he responds to this loving touch.

The Arms

Move from the abdomen to the arms, working first one arm and then the other. With both hands, one on each side of the arm, wring down the arm and back up again. You are using this stroke to circulate the blood flow. Let both your hands glide down the arm from the shoulder to the hand, and then use a gliding stroke back up toward the heart. Repeat these gliding strokes three times. Hold the mother's hand in your hands, letting your fingers stretch the palm, pulling from the center as your thumbs rest on top of the hand.

Effleurage the inside of the arm from the wrist up to underarm area and back to the wrist; repeat at least three times. Using both hands, petrissage down the arm from the shoulder to the wrist and back up; repeat twice. To complete this arm, use feather strokes from the shoulder to the wrist and back up to the shoulder; repeat three times. Move to the other arm and follow the same routine.

The Legs

Standing to the side of the mother, use both your hands to make very light, long sweeping strokes up and down one leg. Sweep with a gliding effleurage stroke from the top of the foot up the front of the legs to the hip. Roll under the leg, and glide from the back of the thigh to the calf to the bottom of the foot. Your touch should be gentle and steady, with absolutely no deep pressure and no held or static pressure on any one spot.

Please refer back to the section "Avoid Some Massage Techniques" in this chapter for a reminder on certain massage techniques you should not use, especially on the lower legs.

> ### Pregnancy Weight Gain
> The weight gain a woman experiences during pregnancy is not only from the growth of the fetus. Amniotic fluid, which protects the baby from shock and regulates temperature, causes some of the weight gain, and so does the placenta, which feeds the growing baby and produces needed hormones.

Back at the ankle, use both hands and circle the pads of your fingers along either side of the shinbone up to the knee. Use a very easy, gentle touch at the knee, circling around the kneecap, but never pressing directly on it. Then, with both your hands, use your fingers to very gently move up the underside of the calf from the ankle to the knee. From the top side of the knee, circle and lightly glide up the front of the thigh to the hip with the fingers of both your hands. At the hip, trace a circle, following the shape of the hipbone on to the side of the buttock.

Now gently glide down to the ankle with both hands cupping the leg. At the ankle, glide gently up the entire leg to the hip and back down again. Remember to move easily over the knee area. Lift the leg slightly and pull straight back with an even, steady pull. Glide from the toes to the ankle with both hands.

Glide up and down the foot a number of times using your open hands. Place your thumbs on top of the foot with your fingers on the sole and stretch the skin to the sides. Glide gently over the foot, using your thumbs and fingers to relax all the muscles of the foot. Finish by gently feathering up and down the entire leg before moving to the other leg.

The Back

The best way to work on the back of a pregnant woman is to turn her on her side and place a pillow between her legs. Allow her to turn sideways while you hold up the drape so she can move with privacy. Once she is comfortably lying on her side, position a pillow under her head and another between her legs. These pillows create an extra cushion to help take pressure off the joints. Some mothers need a pillow under their stomachs, too. Adjust the cover so only the mother's back is exposed.

Effleurage the entire back with both hands. Work from the hip to the neck, moving with a steady, even stroke, applying more pressure with each full stroke. Allow your hands to feel for areas of stress and tightness. Focus first on the shoulder area where often you will find a great deal of congestion. Move your fingers in a steady circular motion following the muscles from either side of the spine to the shoulder area. Of course, the side the mother is lying on will miss some of the massage at this time.

The Benefits of Friction

Friction helps to relieve tension in muscles and joints. As the constriction in the muscles is released you will see a red color in the area. This redness represents the increase in circulation as blood flows to the region that was congested.

Starting at the buttock area and moving up to the neck, use your palm to circle the entire area with smooth, deep pressure. Let your hand feel the skin underneath. The receiver's skin will respond to the release as you use your entire hand to press and push along the spine up to the neck and shoulders. Circle and press the neck and shoulder area, again feeling for a restriction. Repeat the circle strokes from the buttocks to the neck three times, feathering down the back at the end.

Now circle and press on the hip and buttock with both hands; then, using your fingers, press in and hold the fleshy area at the center of the hip, just below the hipbone. Knead the fleshy area, lifting and wringing, releasing the stress in the muscles there. With a pressing movement using your fingers, press along the side of the leg to the knee and back up to the hip. Place one hand on the shoulder and one hand on the hip, and press and hold at both places for the count of seven. Feather the entire area as you prepare to turn your receiver so that you can work on the other side.

Make sure to remove the pillows from between the legs and under the stomach. Again, hold up the drape to give the receiver privacy as she turns to the other side. Repeat the entire back sequence.

Finishing Up

You have just performed an easy, gentle routine for a pregnant woman. This massage or variations of this massage may be used throughout an entire pregnancy. During labor, if the mother permits, you can modify this routine, perhaps working only the back. After delivery and during postpartum recovery, massage is a wonderful tool that can expedite the mother's healing. Massage between partners is an expression of love and compassion that can be shared from the beginning of pregnancy and throughout their lives. Celebrate touching with compassion. Incorporate massage as an essential tool in your daily life.

Chapter 13

Infant Massage

The Philosophy of Infant Massage

The importance of touch for a newborn is immeasurable. As the infant enters the world, the safe, warm, protected environment that has enveloped the baby during gestation is stripped away. Now the baby is exposed to the stress of bright lights, loud noises, and open space. Massage is a tool that can help the newborn adapt to stress in a healthful, integrative manner. Just as stress is part of life, so is relaxation.

Infant and parent bonding is essential for proper development of the child. Massage encourages this bonding by forging the link between parents and their infant, providing a powerful supportive foundation. The infant's ability to process sensory, motor, and cognitive input are intrinsic to proper development and growth. Constant touching, talking, cuddling, and stroking of an infant promotes healthy growth and provides positive stimulation for the child's mental and emotional well-being.

> **Online Help**
>
> Visit *www.infantmassageusa.org* for more detailed information about infant massage techniques, benefits, and classes in your area.

Newborns receive many signals as they attempt to cope with life outside the womb. The skin represents the first form of communication—an infant is welcomed into the world through touch. During a typical labor, the contractions of the uterus that thrust the baby forward also stimulate the systems of the infant's body, preparing the baby to function outside of the mother. In essence, labor contractions massage the baby, getting all systems ready to function once the baby is born.

The Necessity of Touch

Touch is imperative from the moment of birth and is a requirement for the continued health and development of the newborn. The more often the newborn is touched, caressed, held, exercised, bathed, and stimulated through any form of loving touch, the better the progression of development for the infant. During the first year of life, babies cannot be touched enough. Touch transmits love and safety to the infant, allowing for enhanced growth as well as proper functioning as the baby grows.

Touch Is a Two-Way Street

The bonding between parents and their infant is essential for all involved, and touch promotes this bond. Parents receive as much by giving soothing touch as the baby who receives it. The love and enjoyment transmitted by touch is unequaled. Loving touch reinforces the importance of the developing relationship between mature adults and their infant.

Siblings and their newborn family member need to bond as well. Involving a sibling in appropriate care of an infant develops a loving, responsible relationship early on. Include your older child in the massage of the new baby, with supervision of course. As the older child gives to the younger, a special sibling bond appears, and massage helps to form this close-knit tie. As siblings massage the newborn they also receive. The satisfaction of bonding with the baby and other involved family members supports the development of self-esteem and love throughout the entire family.

> **Get Siblings Involved!**
>
> Depending upon the age of the siblings, they can be involved in many bonding activities. Older children love to hold, cuddle, hug, and kiss the baby. Assisting in bath time is another bonding tool that is fun for the sibling.

The Effects of Massage on Infants

When you lovingly touch your newborn frequently, you are encouraging strength, intelligence, depth, and emotional security. You are also supporting physiological growth. A baby who is massaged is usually alert and responsive. The infant quickly develops adaptation techniques to his constantly changing and stimulating environment. Contact is the comfort infants crave the most; an infant without nurturing care will not thrive or, at best, will develop poorly. Gentle massage supports the nervous system, allowing the baby to develop a strong immune system as well as good neurological development. Also, a baby's tiny muscles make up only one-fourth of the baby's weight, and massage helps those muscles grow.

Relaxation for Easy Breathing

While infants develop within their mothers, they receive oxygen from the placenta. Upon birth the newborn must adapt immediately to breathing without help. Touch becomes an essential ingredient in helping the infant to relax while learning to breathe deeply on his own. The mother will instinctively hug, kiss, caress, and rock her newborn and constantly rub her baby's back and chest. This massaging assists in the further development of the respiratory system as well as the transition from shallow to deep breathing.

> ### Rocking Has Real Health Benefits!
> Adequate rocking by the mother or other caregiver creates an environment that is reassuring to the baby. Rocking feels like the mother's womb and supports calmness within the baby.

Production of Hormones

Massage supports the endocrine system, which produces hormones that dictate the function of the various organs within the body. The activity of every organ is influenced in part by these hormones. Good touch enables the hormone-producing glands of the endocrine system to function in a state of balance, or homeostasis. Infants who receive massage have greater hormonal support, which in turn increases the activity of their vital organs. Remember, a baby's organs are still learning how to function outside of the womb, so gentle stimulation on a hormonal level is good.

Support of the Nervous System

The central nervous system—the brain and the spinal cord—works with the endocrine system to support homeostasis. Massage assists the central nervous system by encouraging the formation of nerve and brain cells, including the myelin sheath that protects nerve fibers and serves to speed nerve impulses from the brain to other parts of the body. The myelin sheath is not completely formed before the baby is born, but it responds rapidly to tactile stimulation. During infancy, this formation of cells and myelin is very important, and massage contributes to the growth and support of an infant's nerve health.

Relief from Stress and Overstimulation

Being born is stressful, as is surviving outside of the womb. Massaging the newborn and the growing infant helps the baby adapt to the physical world. Entering into the unknown is scary and confusing on any level, but imagine the feelings of a newborn. Massage helps the baby relax from what would otherwise be overstimulation. Touch is essential for the baby to live a healthy life. There is no such thing as too much loving touch.

> ### A Blank Slate
> A baby receives sensory input while in the womb, but the baby's awareness begins upon entry into the physical realm. Everything the baby is exposed to represents a stimulus. As the baby learns to use his sensory organs to interpret these stimuli, all the baby's senses are used to contribute to healthy growth and development.

Stress introduces the opportunity to adjust, to take the new and unknown and make it familiar. However, a baby who has only the constant input of strange and new situations and no reassuring touch may tire and burn out. Massage helps an infant cope and adapt. It gives the baby the time to relax and recharge, enabling the infant to continue to grow. If you introduce massage early in a child's development, he will be better equipped to deal with the stress of life as he grows up.

Techniques for Infant Massage

You use some of the same familiar strokes you learned for adults on babies, too, but your strokes on infants are not as deep as those you use on adults. The "initial touch" you use on adults is called "familiar touch" when you address the infant's body at the beginning of a session. Infants love to be touched and they respond to light, gentle touch once they become familiar with the sensation. You want the baby to become accustomed to massage, not to feel surprised or threatened. The loving massage that you give will bond your relationship in a wonderful way.

The touch that you apply should be light yet firm. Work slowly and easily, keeping contact with the baby through your touch, your voice, and your eyes. Choose a natural unscented, light oil or cream to work on your baby's unclothed areas, staying away from essential oils and oils derived from nuts.

Baby Steps

Infant massage can begin from the moment you hold your baby, with soft easy strokes along your baby's covered back, as your newborn cuddles on your chest. The sooner you touch your newborn the sooner your baby feels secure, loved, and relaxed. Massaging your infant supports the development of your relationship with your child.

Using Familiar Touch

This familiar touch is the first stroke you will apply. It is a gentle stroke that is more of a holding move, using one or both of your hands, depending upon the size of your hands and the baby. Without removing clothes, gently stroke down the baby's front and then back. This is a feathering technique using your fingertips; the touch is light and steady. You will touch the baby from head to toe, talking softly, explaining perhaps what you are doing. This touch will help the infant become familiar with the concept of extended touch. Gently rest your hands on the baby's belly before turning over to do the back.

Using Effleurage and Petrissage

Once the baby has become accustomed to routine touch, you may begin to effleurage. These long, gliding strokes work well on the torso and extremities. With both hands, use your entire palms and the flats of your fingers to apply a light yet firm pressure over the baby's body, stroking down and up.

You will not be kneading the baby's back; however, the baby's arms and legs usually respond well to wringing, milking, rolling, and squeezing. Wringing is very gently twisting and squeezing the arms or legs from the bottom to the top. Do it gently and fluidly. Milking is exactly as it sounds: starting with one hand, apply a gentle pressure from top to bottom of the baby's limbs in a downward motion, followed right away by the other hand beginning where the other hand began and slightly above there. Alternate hands before the first hand is taken off the skin. Rolling is placing the baby's arm or leg between your hands as you actually roll it between them.

Using Circling

This stroke is applied with a slight amount of pressure from your fingertips or palms as they move in small circles. Circling is often applied along the sides of the spine, on the buttocks, around the hips, and on the abdomen. Circling brings you into an area and out again in a continual applied rhythm.

Using Stretching and Pressing

Stretching helps the baby develop a greater range of motion. Newborns are still mimicking their posture in the womb, so easy stretching gives the baby an alternative position to strive for. Gently stretch the baby's limbs into an open position, pulling only as far as the baby will open. You can also stretch the skin by pressing down with your fingers and slightly stretching it away by pulling your fingers to either side. These strokes are good to use as transitions or ending techniques.

> **Keep the Environment Quiet During Massage**
>
> Create a quiet space for you and the infant. The TV and radio are best turned off, and if you play music, choose some that is relaxing with cheerful and gentle sounds. Arrange for massage time to be a quiet playtime for any siblings.

A Simple Routine

To perform the massage you can either hold the baby on your knees or place the baby on a pad on the floor or in a crib, whichever is most comfortable for both of you. Regardless, choose a space that allows you to keep your back straight while you move your body in rhythm with your strokes. Make sure the room is warm. Your oil should be room temperature, but you should also warm it a bit between your hands before you apply it. Your hands should be clean, your nails trimmed, and your jewelry removed. Undress your baby and wrap him in a towel.

Try to establish a regular routine with your infant. Give your baby time to digest his food, but make sure your baby is comfortable so he does not need to eat while you are in the middle of a massage.

Begin with the Legs and Feet

Babies love to have their feet and legs touched, so this is a good area to begin. Lay your baby face up with his feet near you. Talk to your infant, explaining what you are doing as you unfold the towel from around him. Use a small amount of oil, just enough to allow your hands to glide on your baby's legs. Hold the right foot with your left hand and gently stroke up the leg from the ankle to the thigh and back down again, repeating three times. Place your hand under the leg and glide up and back on the underside three times.

Grasp the baby's ankle gently, lift the leg, and use a milking stroke from the ankle to the thigh and back again. Switch hands and, with the same milking stroke, work the thigh to the hip and buttock and back to the ankle again. If your baby likes this stroke, do it again. If the infant seems fidgety, complete only one cycle. The baby will become more accustomed to this stroke the more often you massage your infant.

Now bring both your hands to one side of the baby's right leg. Beginning at the ankle, use a wringing motion, moving each hand in the opposite direction as you wring up the leg to the thigh and back down again. Repeat. As you twist back and forth be gentle—this is a wringing, not a friction, movement. Lift the leg up and wring to the thigh and gently effleurage down to the foot.

Happy Feet

The foot is one of the best places to massage on an infant. In fact, you could just massage the feet and the baby would relax. Notice how calm the baby becomes as you hold the right foot in your hands and gently stretch the sole of the foot with your thumbs.

With your fingers resting on the top of the foot, let your thumbs meet at the center of the bottom of the foot. Stretch the skin out to the sides and back again. Continue this stretching down the entire surface to the heel.

Cup the foot between both your hands and gently wring the foot, up and down. Using your thumbs make gentle circles around the ankle and circle onto the top of the foot. Slowly squeeze each toe very gently and then press your thumbs into the ball of the foot. Let your thumbs make walking movements along the ball of the foot. Rest both your hands on the foot, feeling the heat from your palms permeate the foot. Repeat this sequence on the left leg and foot, starting with the wringing motion from the ankle to the thigh.

Next, bend each leg by holding the foot at the ankle and bending the knee. Gently stretch out each leg and bend it again. Begin to press and stretch the legs at opposite times as though the baby is riding a bicycle. Now bend both legs at the same time and stretch those legs out once more. Gently roll each leg between your hands from the ankle to the hip and back again.

Chest and Abdomen

The natural progression from the legs is to move up to the abdomen and chest region. Massaging the abdomen helps with digestion and elimination; massaging the chest helps stimulate the lungs and the heart. The baby should be more relaxed now, especially if you have continued to talk quietly, letting him know what you are doing.

Begin with a very gentle press on your baby's belly, turning this press into a circle that moves from the right to the left. Continue circling clockwise on your baby's stomach with steady, gentle movements.

What Is Failure to Thrive?

Failure to thrive is an infant's inability to grow and flourish. Traditionally, this condition was linked to inadequate pituitary production, especially the growth hormone. Later studies proved that the insufficient hormone production from the pituitary gland is caused by the lack of human touch. Massage is one of the tools that can be used to correct this lack.

Use your fingers and gently trace the outline of a circle from the right side of the abdomen up to the waist, across the belly, and down the left side. Continue to make slow, deliberate kneading strokes inside this circle following in the same clockwise direction. The pressure here is still gentle but steady as you move around the area of the colon and small intestines. Eventually you will end up at the bellybutton, where you press gently and hold for the count of five.

Place both your hands on the baby's chest, with your palms on the belly and your fingers resting on the rib cage. This is a very comforting position because the pressure from your warm, loving hands gives the baby a feeling of security. Gently press your hands out to the baby's sides, stretching and pressing as you move. Finally, circle down the sides to the belly and back up the center to the chest again. Repeat.

Hands and Arms

Effleurage down the chest and up again as you move your hands across the baby's shoulders and down the arms. Bring both hands back to the shoulders and glide down both arms to the fingers. Repeat this stroke again, gently stretching the baby's arms out straight. You may glide and stretch two or three times as you are opening the baby's arms with this move.

Respect the Baby's Wishes

If your baby pulls away and wraps her arms close to her chest, do not force the arms apart or away from this protective stance. Some babies do not like having their arms massaged. Simply massage the baby's arms in this hugging posture. As the baby becomes more familiar with the touch, she will open her arms.

Now lift the right arm and milk from the hand to the underarm area. Gently stroke with your fingers under the arm, moving your fingers toward the heart. Squeeze and twist in a wringing stroke up the arm and down; repeat. Lightly stroke down both sides of the arm to the fingers and gently open the hand. Next, stroke with your fingertips on the inside of the baby's hand as you rest the hand in your other palm. Use your thumb and index finger to press each tiny finger, gently. Do not pull the fingers! Make small circles around both sides of the baby's wrist before you finish by stroking the top of the hand. Repeat this process on the other arm.

The Back

Place your baby on his stomach with his legs stretched toward you. He may be on a flat, soft surface or across your legs; whichever both of you are comfortable with. Use a soft effleurage stroke, moving down the back, over the buttocks, and up the back again. Place your hands horizontally across the baby's back, one hand leading the other. Use a soft effleurage stroke and gently glide down the back, over the buttocks, and up to the neck several times.

Place both hands on the back with your fingers pointed at the shoulders. Glide up to the shoulders, along the side of the neck, and down the backs of the arms. Repeat this stroke. Now place both hands on the back and stroke with the entire hand down the back to the heels, using firm light pressure. Repeat.

Bring both hands onto the back and circle with your fingertips over the entire back area. Then gently knead the buttocks with the palms of your hands in small circles. Stroke each of your hands down the leg to the heel, gently holding the heels. Finish with soft feather touches, staying in contact with your baby while you softly stroke from the neck to the feet. Place both hands on the back and rest.

The Face

Turn the baby face up, resting both your hands ever so lightly on your baby's head as you look into his eyes and talk to him. Softly stroke down the sides of the skull to the jaw, bringing your fingers to the chin. If your baby likes this movement, repeat it two or three times. Play peekaboo by placing your open hands lightly over your baby's face, then use your fingers to stretch the skin softly across the forehead. Gently circle with your fingertips along the sides of the forehead.

Ear Info

The earlobe is a point used in reflexology and other pressure methods for relaxation. All babies know this innately—a baby will stroke her ear when she is tired and needs comfort. The gentle stroking of the lobe triggers the nervous system to release chemicals that help relax the body.

Using your thumbs and index fingers, pinch along the jaw up to the cheekbones. Place your thumbs on either side of the nose and stroke up along the side of the nose and out across the cheekbones. Stroke across the cheekbones and up to the ears, letting your fingers brush lightly on the ears. Place your thumbs on the inside of the earlobes and your index finger on the fleshy outside. Easily and lightly stroke down the lobes, squeezing them between your thumbs and index fingers. Stroke down the earlobes several times, and watch how relaxed the baby becomes.

Stretches

The best way to finish the massage is to perform some easy stretches with your baby. The infant is already lying face up, so hold the baby's hands in your hands and stretch the arms across the chest, and then open them. Continue to bring the arms in and across, and open, perhaps singing or talking as you make exercise play. Carefully stretch the arms up over the head, out to the sides, and then down, essentially moving in a semicircle.

Next, hold your baby's ankles in your hands and stretch one leg over the other across the abdomen, repeating several times. Now gently stretch the legs down away from the torso in a straight line before pushing the legs up to a bent-knee position. Repeat this move twice, making sure your baby is enjoying the stretching. Using gentle effleurage, stroke across your baby's body from shoulder to hip, continuing down the leg and off the foot. Press your hands easily into your baby's chest and hold. Thank your baby for a wonderful experience.

> **Kids and Touch**
>
> Massage is a form of holding, and until puberty children need to be stroked and held by their parents. "I love you" is best said through touch until the child reaches about the age of twelve.

Massage and the Older Child

Once you have established a massage routine with your baby, it is easy to continue with this as she grows. Loving touch becomes a special part of your baby's day whether it is enjoyed after a bath or as part of a diaper-change or bedtime routine. All babies need comfort and care, especially throughout the first two years of life. From the moment she wakes up to the ritual at sleep time, loving comforting touch is crucial to your child's health and well-being. Massage can also help the older child to relax not only muscles but feelings as well.

If you want to find out how your older child is feeling, provide a safe comfort zone through massage. This is a zone where the child can share feelings. Older children have fears that they often do not know how to express. They may harbor resentment, anger, worry, fear, or a sense of abandonment. Loving touch creates the safe space needed to let out those fears and release tension.

Modifying the Infant Massage Routine

You have established a massage routine with your newborn that you can change to fit your growing child. All the massage strokes you used when your child was an infant still apply but now they must cover a larger area because your child's limbs and torso have grown. So you must adjust your movements to compensate. When you glide use a more sweeping technique to carry you along the longer limbs. The circles can be larger, too, but the pressure is still gentle. Your child is old enough to give you feedback, so be sure to ask what feels good and what does not.

> For more information on childhood massage, look for Tina Allen's book *A Modern-Day Guide to Massage for Children* (Blue Miso Books, 2014) and classes at *www.liddlekidz.com/liddle-kidz-childrens-massage.html*.

Teach your child to circle on her abdomen, which will help her to get rid of tension in the stomach and help with elimination. Now that the child is older, teach her a stretching routine that she can do whenever she likes:

- Reach for the sky and bend to the ground.
- Stretch your arms out to the side and bend sideways; then stand tall and twist.
- Stand on one foot as you bend your other leg at the knee, lifting the foot off the floor, learning to balance.

- Lie on the floor with knees bent and make bicycle movements, pushing first one leg and then the other.
- Hug yourself, stretching your folded arms up to your chin and back to your chest.

Finish by teaching your child to stroke her own earlobes. Show her how to gently stroke along the lobe with the index finger, supporting with the thumb.

From birth through childhood, massage can be used to promote healthy emotional and physical growth. Start early, and encourage everyone in your family to become involved with the loving gift of massage.

Chapter 14
Sports Massage

The Concept of Sports Massage

Whatever you do with your body, at whatever age you are, if you are physically active you will benefit from sports massage. Sports massage improves circulation and helps provide greater endurance. Sports massage also helps prevent injury by warming up the muscles and creating length in the fascia. This type of massage also helps repair injuries caused by repetitive use.

Sports massage can be administered during training for an event, before an event, and after an event. Sports massage protocol involves certain massage strokes, stretches, and injury-prevention exercises tailored to the sport and muscles used in the activity. After massage, athletes may choose to use cold or hot compresses as well.

The Origins of Sports Massage

Sports massage has a multinational history. Although the idea of massage specifically for athletes originated in Greece, the techniques have a close connection with those used in Swedish massage. These techniques were further refined by sports trainers in Russia.

Athletes may be competitive in the professional arena or they may be more casual, such as when athletes compete against themselves. By helping competitors stay injury-free, sports massage gives them an edge over other participants. Sore muscles recover more quickly and become stronger and suppler when massaged. A massage before an event is a great way to warm up muscles, preparing the competitor for whatever activity she may be undertaking. Actually, sports massage could be renamed competitors' massage, because this describes who the massage is really for.

The Effects of Sports Massage

The massage geared toward the physically active has tremendous benefits. The obvious effect of sports massage is better performance, regardless of what it is you actually do with your body. Sports massage helps you reach your peak physically by improving your circulation while keeping your muscles strong and flexible. Improved circulation reduces your chances of injury and allows for better overall movement.

Sports massage also warms up the muscles beyond whatever stretching you may do. It warms up the connective tissue (fascia), as well as the deeper muscles. Working on the belly of the muscle promotes the distribution of oxygen throughout the entire muscle. Oxygen energizes the muscle, and waste products that interfere with muscle function are encouraged to leave the body through the blood and the lymph system.

Sports massage also helps strengthen and tone your muscles by keeping them free of trigger points and taut bands of fibers. The soothing effect massage has on the nerves helps promote a state of well-being, allowing you to perform at your best. As your nerves relax, tension begins to release, giving you a chance to visualize yourself as a winner. Whether you are playing a sport for a national team, building a house, dancing onstage, or competing in a high school sport, your performance is important.

Avoiding Ischemia

The condition known as ischemia, a deficiency of blood to a particular area, is a common side effect of physical exercise. This obstruction of blood flow causes trigger points, which in turn cause pain or spasms in the muscle. If these spasms and soreness are not treated, they can develop into chronic sites of pain. Left untreated, extreme ischemia can even cause tissue death. Massage is an effective way to virtually eliminate this issue.

Sports massage works through the application of certain strokes by first relaxing the nerve receptors and then invigorating these same receptors through a different application of strokes. Depending upon the athlete's need, the massage can be both relaxing and stimulating, or only one of these. Sports massage is generally provided in a short, timed session that provides energy before an event or brings relaxation after an event. The improvement in soft tissue through this type of massage allows for better and longer performance, with less chance of injury and quicker recovery.

Techniques for Sports Massage

The various techniques employed in sports massage are derived from Swedish massage. The basic strokes are effleurage, petrissage, friction, stretching, and pressing, which you learned about in Chapter 5. These strokes are applied depending upon what the athlete needs from the massage. In this chapter you will learn which strokes to apply, for how long, and with what intensity, all in the context of sports massage.

Using Effleurage Strokes

Effleurage is the gliding stroke that flows over the body of the recipient. You use this stroke to smooth and warm up the body before you move in deeper. Remember to push toward the heart first and then pull back. You can see in Figure 34 how your hands should rest. Your palms should be flat on the contours of the body, with your wrist extended, not stiff or flexed.

Effleurage may also be applied by making circles over the area you are working, which is a deeper movement. This circular stroke flushes out toxins and increases circulation in a smaller area. You may effleurage with either long, gliding strokes or tighter circles; either one helps prepare the receiver for all other massage work.

Keep Your Hands Loose

One of the biggest mistakes made by someone applying massage is to use her hands and fingers incorrectly. Do not bend at the joints. Your fingers should not bend in a sharp angle from your hands, and your hands should not bend in a sharp angle from your wrists. Hold your hands so that they flow into your arms, and keep your wrists flexible.

Using Petrissage Strokes

Following effleurage you might introduce the kneading application of petrissage. With this stroke you lift the tissue into your palm and knead or squeeze to release tension. This method works on the back and the thigh, while smaller areas are more easily worked by using your fingers and thumbs.

Fulling is a petrissage technique that works well in sports massage. For this stroke you knead, with the limb held between the hands, rolling it backward and forward. Practice the fulling stroke on your thigh by placing both hands on either side of the thigh muscle and pushing the muscle up in the middle before stretching away on either side.

Skin rolling is another petrissage move that works well in sports massage. This stroke is applied by lifting the tissue up between your fingers and thumbs as you compress the tissue. Roll the skin between your fingers using both hands as you move along the area, lifting, pressing, and rolling in one continuous motion. This technique may be painful at first so remember to ask your receiver if she is comfortable with your touch. This rolling helps loosen the fascia, connective tissue, and helps release adhesions.

Petrissage also increases the blood flow and moves toxins up for release. It also helps release hormones that relieve pain, and it stimulates the nervous system as well. The release of tension with petrissage is very effective because it reaches the deeper layers of muscle and fascia. Muscle soreness and stiffness are reduced and sometimes eliminated with petrissage.

Using Friction Strokes

Friction applies heat to the underlying muscle while moving the top layer of skin over the deeper layers. Friction helps improve circulation within the tendons and ligaments, which are areas that generally do not receive much blood flow. The initial friction stroke is applied with your hands flat down on the body. Your hands move back and forth in two straight lines passing each other in a continued movement along the surface being worked. The movement is steady with an increase in speed as you become accustomed to the body underneath.

Friction of the arm or leg is done by rolling or wringing the area between both hands in opposite directions. This is cross-fiber friction. You may friction the forearm or calf in this manner by bending the recipient at the elbow or knee and wrapping both your hands around the limb. Figure 35 shows you how to position your hands and fingers to wring the muscles of the calf.

Think of cross-fiber movements as small bites working their way across the muscle, as opposed to smooth, gliding movements up and down the muscle fibers or in-and-down pressing movements. Cross-fiber friction can be applied all over the body, including the extremities. Place your fingers on the area and firmly press in a back-and-forth motion.

Using Stretching

As a massage therapist, you can both stretch the receiver and teach her how to stretch. Passive stretching by you helps to extend the muscle tissue without the receiver participating. You apply gentle pressure to allow the muscle to stretch a tiny bit farther than it could without your assistance. Effleurage provides some of this stretch because it loosens connective tissue. You may assist further with a simple guidance of the body part in the direction of the stretch.

In another form of assisted stretching, active contract/relax, the receiver is an active participant. You allow the recipient to press or pull a muscle or group of muscles that you are holding. For example, hold the receiver's arm out straight in one hand and ask her to press down on your resisting hold; then reverse your hold and ask the receiver to press up into your hand. This type of stretch assists in developing strength and flexibility of the muscles as opposer muscles alternately learn how to contract, then relax.

Finally, encourage your athlete to follow a full regimen of stretching post-workout as well as warming up the muscles before an event or activity.

> ### Warming Up Is Not the Same as Stretching
>
> Warming up a muscle is very different from stretching. During warm-up, the athlete should mimic in a slower and less powerful way the same moves necessary for the behavior or activity she will be performing, such as walking on a treadmill before running or swinging the arms while pretending to hit a tennis ball (but without a racket) or jumping jacks before a track meet. It is important to allow one's temperature and circulation to increase before moving into any activity, including stretching.

Stretching helps to relax and release sore muscles and fascia, allowing for quicker recovery. Stretching also helps relaxation by increasing all soft tissue flexibility and mobility. In the more relaxed state, both the flow of blood and oxygen improves as well.

Using Static Compression

This method of massage is used to increase circulation and encourage the relaxation of the muscle fibers that may have become taut bands. Pressing, or compression, helps to warm up the muscle, which helps an athlete prepare for activity. Position the palm of your hand or the elbow on the muscle that needs attention and apply pressure directly onto the belly of the muscle in a steady rhythmic motion. Coordinate the compression with deliberate relaxation on the slow exhale of the recipient and release the compression as she breathes in again. Place your other hand on top of the pressing hand to assist in the application of pressure. Remember not to bend at the wrist but to keep the hand loose. Press through the area using your body weight and not your own muscle strength. If your recipient's muscles are very dense, the palm might not provide enough pressure—in those cases, use your forearm.

If you encounter a muscle in spasm, apply even pressure without moving as you encourage the recipient to bring attention and relaxation to this area. Keep your hand on the spasm for a count of ten and then with a coordinated exhale, release the pressure. The compression and release will help reduce the spasm in the muscle, will unlock the contracted muscle fibers, and will promote local circulation.

Using Tapping

Tapping as part of a sports massage is performed with the sides of your hands or your fingers along the affected area. It is an invigorating technique that stimulates blood and oxygen flow, and is used to provide added energy, generally before an event. Tapping provides a toning effect that helps to warm up the muscles.

When to Massage Athletes

The application of sports massage depends upon the needs of the individual athlete. Typically, it is most effective when used during training as well as during competition; before an event, after an event, and as maintenance long-term.

During Regular Training

During training, athletes work to strengthen muscles for endurance, power, coordination, and injury prevention. Massage enhances the athlete's performance and familiarizes the receiver to sports massage techniques. The technique you use for the athlete in training is the same routine as any Swedish massage, with an emphasis on areas of the body that experience added stress due to the particular exercise, sport, or job the athlete participates in.

If the athlete is willing to continue massage even when not competing, she will reap its long-term benefits. Maintenance massage keeps the muscles and fascia healthy while dealing with any chronic soreness or pain.

Before an Event

Pre-event massage is used as an additional warm-up, providing an edge to the performance of the athlete. This massage is styled to provide stretch and movement by encouraging the flow of blood and oxygen to the muscles and loosening connective tissue. The athlete's body will perform better due to the improved flexibility of the muscles and fascia. With improved muscle function, the athlete can perform better, faster, stronger.

Often overtraining can cause overly tight muscles, trigger points, restriction, and also mental tension. A ten-minute massage applied thirty minutes before an event will not only relieve tight, tense muscles but it will also invigorate all the athlete's senses, providing a positive degree of readiness. Before an event do not use deep pressure and do not stay too long on one spot. The idea is to give broad added support physically, mentally, and emotionally through your massage.

Your Body Can Heal Itself

Your body works to stay in a state of balance, constantly working toward homeostasis. The trauma of damaged tissue sets a process in motion to let the body heal itself. Inflammation is the body's way of saying slow down and take a break. If the body heeds the message, regeneration can occur.

After an Event

Massage after an event is a powerful way to deal with the aftereffects of a rigorous routine. The muscles in the participant's body have been pushed to the limit, causing the muscle tissue to swell. There may be soreness and inflammation depending upon the level of trauma the muscles have sustained. Such discomfort following exercise responds well to massage, and a thirty-minute massage after the event will help with these issues.

After an activity, sports massage helps to restore the muscles to their normal condition and helps the body to heal itself. The muscles that have experienced contraction and spasm begin to relax during massage as the toxins are pushed from the body. The high mental tension the performer maintained during the event is also released during massage as the body begins to relax. Percussive massage tools such as the MyoBuddy can be used to speed post-activity recovery and muscle relaxation.

Postevent becomes postrecovery as the body moves toward repair. If muscle soreness does not dissipate, continue working with the athlete on a weekly basis, addressing specific issues through a longer massage. As you work toward releasing soreness, your massage will teach the receiver's muscles to loosen and stretch naturally. Regular sports massage locates and removes chronic issues and helps the receiver become more aware of the needs and requirements of his or her body.

The more the participant understands the benefit of long-term massage, the better equipped the athlete will be to consistently perform well. Sports massage maintenance improves all aspects of the athlete's life by helping the athlete develop a pattern of injury-free living. Regular massage supports the heavy demands of the athlete's performance and enhances her ability to maintain strength and endurance.

Routines for Sports Massage

The routine for sports massage depends upon the athlete and what phase—training, pre-event, postevent—you are dealing with. Massage given during training can be primarily a maintenance technique. Massage given before an event is energizing, while a massage given after the event is relaxing and healing. Generally, sports massage is administered with little or no oil and the receiver stays clothed. Of course, any massage may be given this way.

Pre-Event Warm-Up for the Back of the Body

Given before a sports event, this massage provides the benefits of a warm-up and at the same time invigorates the mind and body, stimulating the systems to a state of complete readiness.

1. To begin, have your receiver lie facedown, and then apply strong effleurage strokes in great sweeping movements over her back from the base of the spine up to the shoulders, and back around. Remember to move your body in a rocking motion as you apply these strokes, moving in toward the receiver on the up stroke and back from the receiver on the down stroke.
2. Repeat this effleurage a number of times, using smooth, steady, firm pressure. Listen to your hands while you work.
3. Now apply compression on the back with a rhythmic pumping, moving up the back along the spine to the shoulders. Repeat this three or four times, pumping smoothly over the surface of the back. If the receiver indicates she has spasms in this area, press down on and hold the region (do not pump), and then release upon exhale after the count of ten.
4. With your hands or just your fingers, use a tapping motion from the receiver's waist to the shoulders and down the back, providing stimulation to the muscles.
5. Next, knead over the buttocks as demonstrated in Figure 36, and then continue down the legs with a gliding stroke.
6. Apply an effleurage stroke up the legs from the ankles to the buttocks and back to the ankles. Using a friction stroke, start at the ankle and wring up the calf to the back of the knee and down to the ankle, repeating three or four times. At the top of the knee begin with a circling pressure stroke, and stroke up the leg to the hips and buttocks. Using petrissage, knead the hips and buttocks before turning the receiver over.

Pre-Event Warm-Up for the Front of the Body

1. With the recipient lying on her back, start the front massage of the arms and legs. Begin on the right arm and effleurage from the wrist to the shoulder and back again, three times.
2. Apply a rolling stroke along the arm, lifting it when necessary to reach all parts of the arm.
3. Bend the arm at the elbow and wring it from the wrist to the elbow and back again. With both your hands, stretch the right hand on both sides.

4. Now, starting with the recipient's arm at her side, parallel to the body, use both your hands to carefully stretch the arm out to the side, and up alongside the recipient's ear, then back through to the recipient's side. Repeat on the left arm.

5. Move to the left leg and effleurage in long sweeping strokes up from the ankle to the hip and down, three to five times.

6. Then wring up from the ankle to the knee, and repeat three times.

7. Next, lift and roll the thigh muscles up to the hips using a kneading stroke, and repeat three times.

8. Move back to the recipient's feet and, using both hands, stretch the left foot on the top and the bottom. After the stretch, rest both hands on the top of the left foot with your thumbs reaching across the sole. Wring up and down the foot, as demonstrated in Figure 37.

9. Repeat your massage on the right leg starting with effleurage from the ankle to the hip, and ending with wringing the right foot.

10. Complete the leg massage by tapping each leg from the ankle to the hips.

Postevent Massage

It is best to provide massage as soon as possible following an event, because waste products may have built up during an activity, and these can cause sore, painful, and sensitive muscles. Postevent massage helps to prevent stiffness and fatigue, and helps the athlete to relax.

1. Begin with the receiver lying on her stomach, and effleurage the entire back from the waist to the shoulders and back to the waist.

2. Then gently glide up both the recipient's arms, one at a time, from the hands to the neck and back to the hands. Repeat three times on each arm before moving to the legs.

3. Now glide up the thigh from the back of the knee over the buttocks and down through the hips back to the knee.

4. Finally, effleurage from the ankle to the back of the knee and back down to the ankle. Repeat three times, with each glide becoming deeper. Then move on to the other leg.

As your hands glide over the body, can you feel what areas are tense? More than likely the legs hold most of the tension, followed by the back or neck, but this depends on the activity that was just completed. The next part of the massage is designed to relieve this tension in the legs.

1. Begin with fulling the hamstrings by placing both your hands on either side of the left thigh, just above the back of the knee. Press in to push up the muscle, and then stretch out the skin to the sides. Perform this fulling technique up the back of the leg to the top of the thigh, and repeat moving down to your starting position, just above the back of the knee.

2. Carefully knead along the entire back of the thigh from the knee to the buttock and back again. Stroke gently over the back of the knee and continue kneading the entire calf muscle, if this move feels fine to the recipient.

3. Then, using friction, pinch and roll the calf from the ankle to the knee, stopping just below the soft area behind the knee. Use this pinch-and-roll friction down the calf and back up to the knee, repeating this stroke twice more.

4. Wring up the left leg from the ankle to the knee, stroke over the knee, and knead up to the top of the thigh. Standing to the left side of the person makes this move easy.

5. Now place your hands on the left buttock, one hand on top of the other, with the heel of your palm pressing into the buttock. Press, release; press, release, and press and hold, feeling the buttock relax.

6. Next, stand at the recipient's feet, hold the left leg by the calf, and bend the leg into the buttock as far as the leg will easily go. Do not force the stretch. Slowly release the leg and repeat the entire procedure on the right leg, starting with the fulling of the right thigh.

Pain Is Communication

After an event, massage should not cause more pain to muscles that are already sore. If after the initial touch the receiver complains of pain, then move away from that area. Application of specific pressure too soon after a sporting event will only cause more stress, and will not allow the muscle to fully relax.

This basic postevent routine can be used on any area of the body that is feeling stress from the activity. Make sure the recipient drinks plenty of water to flush out the toxins and metabolic waste that your massage work released from the muscles and other organs. In addition to releasing built-up toxins, the postevent massage jump-starts the blood and lymph flow. Remind your receiver to breathe during the massage, and stretch after it is over.

Understanding Sports Injury

Dedicated athletes often work in pain, and it becomes part of their lives. Athletes will not generally stop training and competing, but instead make the conscious choice to work through the pain. You may want to explain how ignoring pain can lead to further challenges and greater impairment if a true injury occurs. Pain is information and should not be ignored. Once you have presented these ideas and have made your position clear, the choice to continue is then the responsibility of the recipient. Allow the performer to make an educated decision from your information, as you remain clear that your intention is to provide healing as needed.

Overloading

Athletes often try to improve their performance by training with a technique known as overloading. The idea is that the more you do the more you challenge your cardiovascular system and muscles, and the more you improve your performance. The other part of this idea is that the body must rest and recover in order for you to continue reaching for added challenge. Sometimes athletes do too much too fast and do not allow their bodies sufficient time to recover between challenges. As a result, they end up with overuse injuries.

The damage caused by overuse may result in a variety of injuries to the soft tissue of the body. Massage is an important tool in the repair of this damage. Muscle soreness is the most frequent complaint and is associated with a small degree of pain and perhaps spasms. Effleurage, compression, and petrissage are good techniques to help remedy this type of injury.

Strains and Sprains

Strains and sprains are injuries often caused by quick movements or by muscles that are acutely overstressed. When soreness that is ignored creates shifts in the way the body is used, this can lead to muscle substitution and to non-neutral joint movements. Then when the area is quickly lengthened or overloaded, the fibers can tear or separate. When such an injury occurs in a muscle, it is called a strain; when it occurs in a ligament, it is called a sprain. The tearing of tissue and the resulting scarring can be painful. Whichever injury is sustained, initial swelling and pain must subside somewhat before massage can be used. Friction massage is helpful in working with the misaligned fascia or scar that forms under the skin as the tissue repairs itself.

Sports massage can help anyone who is active. If you use your body for more than sitting, you can benefit from all aspects of this type of massage. Children can benefit from shorter sessions, because often they cannot remain still for the full sessions. Anyone you know who needs some rest and restoration can benefit from sports massage.

Chapter 15
Massage and Aging

The Principles of Elder Massage

Based on information from the U.S. Census Bureau, in 2010, people eighty-five years old and over are the fastest growing group of people in the country. While many of the elderly population are active and healthy, maintaining their independence longer, the oldest of the old do begin to fail. People older than eighty-five may face a decline in health as well as loss of independence and loss of their partners. More women than men reach the oldest age group, and so many elderly women are living alone without partners. This circumstance can turn into isolation, which is a threat to the health and well-being of an elderly person. Massage is a way to combat this threat.

> ### How Many Are There?
>
> According to the U.S. Administration on Aging, there were approximately 44 million people in the United States over the age of sixty-five in 2013. They represented about 14 percent of the total U.S. population.

The Social Connection

Massage for the elderly not only provides physical healing, it also provides the opportunity for the recipients to interact with someone else, lifting them out of their isolation. Anyone who is confined, whether through physical limitations or living arrangements, can benefit from the time spent with another person before, during, and after a massage. Before a massage session, the receiver generally shares any physical concerns that she may be experiencing at the time. During the massage the recipient may feel more relaxed, more in touch with his body, and certainly more alive. After a massage session, the communication gates are fully open as the receiver basks in the enjoyment of caring touch and loving concern.

The Effects of Massage on the Elderly

Touch is important during any phase of life, as expressed by Ashley Montagu, the late pioneer and revered expert in the field of touch, who wrote: "It is especially in the aging that we see touching at its best as an act of spiritual grace and a continuing human sacrament." With the loss of so many senses and functions as one ages, the need for healing touch is crucial. Our elder community needs, wants, and deserves the compassionate touch that massage can provide.

> **Rethink Aging**
>
> Too often the concept of aging brings to mind isolation, illness, and death. You can help an elder stay in touch with not only the exciting aspects of growing older but also with the joy of being touched. Massage for the elder population is important for their emotional, physical, mental, and spiritual well-being.

With aging, the elasticity of the skin is affected. Wrinkles and spotting often appear, along with dryness and a change in pigment. As people age, their receptors for touch become less sensitive, especially the nerve endings in their palms. Informed touch stimulates the skin and helps keep it supple and alive, while at the same time reinforces the tone of the muscles that lie under the connective tissue that provide support.

Some of the benefits of massage that particularly affect the elderly include:

- Stimulates the appetite
- Releases hormones
- Improves sleep
- Reduces joint pain
- Relieves swelling
- Stimulates circulation
- Lowers blood pressure
- Supports elimination

The application of massage is helpful for virtually all of the many needs an elder has.

Seniors Give Back

Studies have shown that elders feel just as good giving a massage as receiving one. Giving a massage says, "I care enough to find out about you." When a younger member of the family receives a massage from a grandmother or grandfather, the message is, "You are important to me." Often children do not perceive the elders in the family as connecting with them in a real and meaningful way. So teach yourself to give a massage to your grandchildren or other loved ones. Organize your group of friends and have a massage party, or learn self-massage. Loving contact is for everyone, and massage is a special time together that allows communication on many levels.

When Massage Is Okay

Massage and aging for the most part are complementary. Massage can discourage the rapid onset of illness and aging by helping the elderly to remain strong. Working on the muscles of an older person helps that person to have more control of his body; the recipient becomes less stiff and has fewer aches and pains. Better muscle control leads to better coordination and dexterity, both of which tend to decline with age. Many people seem to forget that touch is therapeutic. Whatever stage of life you are in, massage has a place in your wellness program.

When Massage Is Not Okay

Today, doctors and other health providers accept and applaud the concept of compassionate touch on all populations, especially the elderly. But it is always important to make sure the doctor knows about any additional health measures a patient is taking, including massage. Although the benefits of massage are plentiful, there are certain medical conditions that signal caution against massaging an elder. The conditions that contraindicate massage are:

- Severe swelling
- Open sores
- Bruises
- Inflammation
- Extreme sensitivity
- Blood clot
- Varicose veins

If an elder suffers from any of these conditions, a full body massage is not appropriate. If none of the conditions indicated are near the face, a gentle face massage may be considered, with a medical practitioner's consent. Easy gliding strokes from the neck up to the forehead will provide comfort, and the elder will benefit from the attention. If it is impossible to give a massage, simply holding hands provides a caring touch full of compassion and will be appreciated.

There are other conditions that require the approval of the receiver's medical practitioner prior to a massage. These are when the elder is:

- Undergoing chemotherapy
- Undergoing radiation therapy
- Recovering from surgery
- Recovering from a stroke
- Recovering from a heart attack
- Living with osteoarthritis

Again, kind touch is healing touch and any form of touching is better than not touching at all. A hand that is held or patted, combined with a hug, while not a massage, still provides caring support.

Techniques and Considerations for Elder Massage

Most of the techniques that you have learned so far are appropriate for massage on an elder. The massage strokes of effleurage, petrissage, pressing, and tapotement are all effective when working with the elderly.

> ## Staying Young
>
> Inside the aging body is a young person, someone who feels that his body seems to have forgotten how to play. Exercise, proper diet, and continued bodywork are part of a lifestyle that allows a person to live life in a continuum rather than feel betrayed as the body fails.

Preparing for an Elder Massage

Elders can become cold easily, so remain mindful of this and keep a light blanket close by. Some older people might not be able to climb onto a massage table. Adapt accordingly, perhaps sitting your elderly recipient sideways on a chair or on a stool pushed up to the bed so the recipient can lean his head on the soft surface. Take your time and improvise with your space until you find what works. You can lower the height of your standard massage table to make it much easier for the receiver to get onto it.

Remember that many members of the senior population move at a slower pace than you do. Use this time to connect with the recipient as she moves slowly to the workspace, and continue your connection afterward when the recipient slowly puts on her shoes. Understand that this is your lesson in patience and learning to wait. Breathe in the moment and enjoy your relationship with the receiver. What a gift to be allowed to slow down and enjoy.

Personalized Contact

Throw away any preconceived stereotypical notions you might have and greet each senior as an individual with his own strengths and frailties. Honor the differences of every person you deal with, regardless of age. There may be certain issues that everyone in the older age group have in common, but remember, everyone is also different!

Understand that not all seniors are frail; many have strong muscles under their visually aging skin. All people hold tension in their body regardless of physical strength. The knots and tightness you find in others may be present with an elder, too. Thin elderly bodies do not necessarily mean weak, brittle bodies. Yes, the bones of elderly people are certainly more brittle and their joints are less flexible than those of younger people, but treat every person as an individual and assume nothing.

Setting Boundaries

Often elders live alone, without many visitors, and have no set schedule. The highlight of their day might be a visit from someone like you who is going to spend quality time with them. By providing a massage and the experience of companionship, you brighten an elderly person's day. You, on the other hand, may have a full schedule. That stop may represent only a part of your busy day. In such circumstances, clarity and good communication are important.

Connections Are Vital

The MacArthur Foundation study on aging inspired Dr. Robert Kahn to cowrite the book *Successful Aging* (Pantheon Books, 1998) where he states that, "We are 'hard-wired,' genetically programmed, to develop and function by interacting with others." Aging people still require family and friends, and without these connections the elderly will have a difficult time surviving.

Be very clear on the amount of time you intend to spend on this visit, keeping in mind that you will, indeed, need more time with the elderly. So plan for it. When you work with an elder the actual time you spend on the massage may be less than the time you work on younger people. However, your elder receiver needs extra time to prepare, to receive, and to recover. In addition, the older person might want to share the interesting points of his life—things that happened recently and things from the past. Give yourself enough time to enjoy the visit, give a quality massage, and still be able to leave when you planned.

A Routine for Senior Massage

Your routine will change according to the person you are working on; however, you can design a blueprint that you can adjust as needed. Consider conducting a shorter session, at least initially. Be aware that an elderly person may not be able to lie in one position for too long at a time. And you may need to provide extra support with certain positions. Also ask how much clothing the receiver wishes to keep on, if any. Some people, no matter what age, prefer to receive massage through the cover, while others feel very comfortable completely in the buff. Use oil that is easily absorbed by the skin and remember to ask whether your recipient prefers scented or not. Finally, make sure the temperature in the room is comfortable for the receiver.

> ### Watch for Spasms
>
> If your receiver is experiencing a muscle spasm, be gentle and deliberate in helping to create relaxation. Guide a gentle inhale and exhale, and focus on bringing relaxation to the area in spasm. Keep your hands gently over the area and provide a distraction around the area in spasm, like gently moving the whole arm or hand. A muscle spasm is a quick, involuntary contraction due to many conditions like chronic dehydration, lack of full movement, and poor posture. Gentle effleurage may help to ease and relax the muscle and connective tissue. Listen to the receiver: if he wants you to leave the area alone, then honor that request.

Back and Shoulder Massage

If the receiver decides that he would like you to work the back and shoulders, and is able to lie facedown for a short period of time, help him into a position that works best for him. Place pillows in areas that need extra support, and cover the recipient with a flannel sheet. Make the receiver as comfortable as possible, and remember to check in to see if he needs to move. Often a short time spent working on the back is as much as your elder recipient can tolerate in that position.

Rest both your hands on the receiver's covered back for a moment. Then pull back the cover, tuck it around the waist, and apply oil with a gentle but firm effleurage stroke on the back, feeling for tension as you glide from the waist to the shoulders and back again. Your hands and fingers will tell you where to hold and press after you finish applying the oil.

Glide along the shoulders and the backs of the arms, moving with a steady, even rhythm.

Return to the areas of tension and gently petrissage between the shoulder blades and around the neck. Remember to use steady, even pressure without digging, and be aware of any fragile areas. Constantly check with the receiver to make sure your pressure is fine. You may be surprised to learn the receiver wants you to press more firmly. Knead along the shoulders and then glide over the entire area again.

Moving On to the Arms and Legs

Remove any pillows or bolsters from under the legs before helping your receiver turn over onto his back. Be supportive; you may have to gently help the recipient up while keeping the drape tucked in for privacy. Carefully assist in any way your receiver needs and then help him to reposition.

Once on the back, place the supports under the legs and perhaps under the neck and shoulders. Effleurage one leg with both your hands. Use firm gliding strokes from the ankle to the knee and then from the knee to the hip. Repeat at least twice before gently kneading the hip area. Again let your fingers be your eyes as you feel where the tension is, while listening to the receiver as well. Glide again over the entire leg and repeat the sequence on the other leg.

> **Keep in Touch!**
>
> Pay attention to the person you are working on as you continue to stay in touch, assessing if the receiver needs to turn or get up. Alter your techniques to fit the body you are working on, and become aware of any limitations.

Work the arms with the same strokes. Start with one arm and effleurage with both your hands from the wrist to the elbow and then from the elbow to the shoulder, using firm gliding movements. Repeat on the other arm. Remember to stroke the joints with a feathering movement. Do not apply pressure. Then knead in the shoulder areas with both hands, using extra caution as you approach the neck. Do not apply any massage to the center of the neck as this area is contraindicated. Gently feather off the shoulders and move to the head.

Strokes for the Face and Head

Stand behind the receiver and gently stroke up the face with both hands from the chin, over the cheeks, pulling off at the forehead. Use circular kneading movements over the entire face, always moving up toward the forehead. Circle your fingers in at the jaw, easing tension that may accumulate in that region. Use feather strokes up the chest, along the sides of the neck, and over the face. Rest your hands, palms flat, over the eyes and hold still.

Using shampoo strokes work the entire top and back of the head, gently lifting the head so you can work the back of the scalp. Rest the head in your hands with your fingertips gently pressing in at the base of the skull. Hold here and breathe. Ask your receiver to breathe with you, slowly and gently.

Keep an Eye on Your Own Aging

As you age, you may find that you feel and function differently. You may feel tight or stiff in the morning, taking a bit more time to begin your day. You can choose to make the most of this experience by making this the time to practice some of the relaxation exercises or self-massage techniques you have learned. This will help you work through the stiffness that your muscles and joints may be experiencing.

Carefully remove your hands and let the receiver know your massage is complete. Give him time to relax and let the massage sink in, then gently say that you will help him get up just to a seated position. Remain in this seated position for a minute or more, then when the elder feels ready to get up, help the receiver stand up and off the table. Remember that elders tend to move a bit slower, so pace your movements with the receiver's. Remember to include some social time at the end of the massage, because talking with the elderly is just as important as your touch.

Touch and the End of Life

You will find that many people do not want to spend time with someone who is in the process of transition to death, because this means confronting their own fear of dying. This is a time when a dying person needs others the most, and if you can overcome your own fears you can provide a powerful gift. Understand that this person needs your sensitivity, your willingness to serve, and your compassionate touch. There are no set rules or regulations here other than to proceed with honor and respect, being mindful of the comfort of the person. Trust that your heart will guide you, and you will be appropriate. Be sensitive to the condition of the person, understanding that change is the constant state of affairs in which this person lives. The wants and needs of the person in transition can fluctuate from moment to moment.

Massage can help the person deal with the emotional stress of the situation as well as the physical discomfort. Approach with love and honesty, giving what you can. Know that compassionate, loving touch is essential during this time, whether it is a foot rub, a shoulder rub, or holding hands.

You are a teacher and a student, giving and receiving simultaneously. An intention to help on any level ensures that you are providing what is needed at any given time. The giving of kind touch breaks down all barriers while the sharing of this touch is splendid.

Chapter 16

Massage Routines for Symptomatic Relief

The Main Goal: Restore Homeostasis

Homeostasis is the internal balance of the body's systems, and stress is the stimulus that upsets that balance. Both physical and psychological stress can upset homeostasis. The internal structure of the body is designed to compensate for most stresses, working constantly to maintain homeostasis; however, at times stress becomes too much for the body to handle. Stress can lead to disease if certain functions within the body are inhibited. Massage helps to reduce this interference by inhibiting the depleting effects of stress while promoting proper system function.

Massage can help with the relief of symptoms of many conditions—if you are not sure, ask a medical practitioner. Most medical advisors recommend some form of massage as a relaxation tool, a stress reliever, and a pain releaser. The important factor in offering massage is your intention. Wanting to give support and care is the key ingredient; you can't go wrong with love in the recipe. Go ahead and give comfort, be it a back rub or a hand massage— you will help bring joy and encouragement to whomever you are massaging.

Causes of Stress

Stress can come from outside the body in the form of physical stimuli like cold, heat, noise, or the lack of oxygen. The body can generally remain in balance, because it is built to deal with these environmental changes. However, at times these physical stressors create more of a response than the body and mind can deal with. For example, too much heat can cause heat stroke or exhaustion as well as a shift in the emotional response, appearing as impatience, even rage.

The continued use of massage as a preventative measure for stress works because it calms the mind as well as the body. Massage works to release the built-up tension in the muscles that causes stiffness and lack of mobility. Relief from these symptoms frees the body to relax and move, and releases the mind from thinking about feeling stiff and sore.

Stress can also come from your social environment, such as the demands of work or family, creating undue stress on the internal environment. Eventually, many stress-related issues can turn into physical complications. Massage can relax the body and mind, help prevent illness, and support good health. In Chapter 8, you learned about the causes of stress and the body's response to them. Here you will learn how to use massage to help treat specific stress-related issues.

Headaches

There are a variety of reasons why you might have a headache:

- Muscle tension and/or trigger points in the neck and shoulders
- A sinus infection
- Jaw clenching
- Susceptibility to migraines
- Eyestrain
- Poor sleep posture
- Chronic slouching or head-forward posture

Massage can help relieve the pain of headaches and sometimes eliminate the cause of headaches. Become aware of your body and understand the warning signs of certain types of headaches. Pay attention to your neck, shoulders, and upper back. If you feel tension and tightness in the muscles in those regions, it is time for a massage. Ideally, you should keep your body fit, limber, and tension-free so that you can stay ahead of the aches and pains.

A Simple Routine to Relieve or Prevent Headaches

1. Place your hands on either side of your face, thumbs in and fingers resting on your temples, and circle gently over your entire forehead up into the hairline; repeat.
2. Circle with your fingers along your jawline from your chin to your ears, work along

the edge and following up with an easy pinching stroke using your thumbs and index fingers.

3. Circle with your fingers on your cheeks, working around the cheekbones up to the sides of your nose; press with your fingertips along the bridge of your nose.

4. Gently pinch along the ridge of your ears from the lobes up to the tops of your ears and back to the lobes again, stroking down the earlobes with your thumbs and index fingers; repeat.

5. Shampoo your head, working your entire head from the back of the skull, along the sides to the top of your head; circle in the ridges at the base of your skull.

6. Circle down the back of your neck, feeling the tight muscles under your fingers; then knead along your shoulders as far as you can comfortably reach and feather off.

The more you practice this simple routine on yourself, the more release of tension you will have in these areas. This will also help relieve sinus headaches, although prevention of sinus-related infection involves managing your diet as well.

Abdominal Issues

Ulcers, gastritis, irritable bowel, and stomachaches are a few of the digestive disorders that may be the result of emotional distress. Nicotine, caffeine, alcohol, spicy foods, and anti-inflammatory medicines can also trigger the formation of ulcers. Some people are genetically predisposed to developing these abdominal problems; however, if they manage to release tension, clean up their diet, and work through their stress, they often do not suffer any symptoms. Proper eating habits and regular practice of stress management work to prevent many of these conditions, too. Not surprisingly, massage is a wonderful antidote as well as a preventative method for dealing with these problems. A full body massage, a chair massage, or a self-massage are all techniques that support the organs of the abdomen and release stress that may be held in that region.

A Simple Routine to Address Abdominal Issues

1. Begin by lying in a comfortable position on your back. You can place a pillow under your knees. Place your hands on your abdomen, just above and on either side of your bellybutton.
2. Notice your breathing. Is it shallow; is it quick? Work to slow your breath, allowing your abdomen to be fully relaxed as it rises and falls with each breath.
3. After a minute or so, move your hands to just above your pelvic bone. Begin slowly working your hands to the right to the edge of your abdomen, then upward to about even with your bellybutton, then take a turn and glide across to the left, then downward and back to the starting point. This right-to-left motion can help elimination. Repeat this three to ten times.
4. Then make a smaller circle inside that radius, and repeat. Continue to breathe slowly, relaxing your neck and chest. Allow the abdominal muscles to completely relax.
5. Place your hands at your pelvic bone again, and glide straight upward to the breastbone (sternum). You may work up to being able to place a pillow under your lower back, slightly arching your back, stretching your abdominal muscles. As you glide upward from the pelvic bone, continue upward along the breastbone, gently along the sides of your neck, then take a "morning stretch" ending with your arms resting over your head on the floor or surface you are lying on.
6. Modify this stretch for the abdominals by grasping the right wrist with the left hand and gently leaning over to the left; hold for three breaths. Finally, return to center to switch to the other wrist.

> **Cellular Respiration**
>
> Respiration also takes place at the cellular level where cells pass gaseous waste to the blood in exchange for oxygen and other nutrients. Oxygen is added to the other components in the cell in a process known as oxidation.

Problems with the Respiratory System

Respiration begins when you inhale through your nose or mouth. The air moves into your lungs where oxygen is passed into the blood and circulated throughout your body. When you exhale, you breathe out the carbon dioxide that your blood has returned to your lungs. This respiration process is continuous.

Polluted air, smoking, exposure to chemicals, and airborne allergens can affect the quality of your breathing. Massage contributes to the health of the respiratory system by supporting the exchange of oxygen and carbon dioxide in the lungs, as well as respiration on a blood and cellular level. Exercise, proper breathing, and a nutritious diet also help maintain the health of your respiratory system.

Often when people experience breathing problems, whether from a cold, allergies, or infection of the nose and sinuses, they find it difficult, if not impossible, to lie facedown while they receive a massage. Ask the recipient if she prefers to lie facedown or with the face turned to the side, or if it is better to turn the entire body to one side as you work on the back. Chair massage is another option for someone with breathing issues. Whatever feels comfortable for the receiver will work. Of course if your massage partner is experiencing painful breathing or shortness of breath, encourage that person to seek medical attention.

Massage During Osteoporosis

It is important for you to know that you can massage someone with osteoporosis (a degenerative bone condition), although you need to modify your technique by using less pressure and slower, easier movements. Diet, nutritional supplements, weight-bearing exercise, and massage all contribute to the prevention of bone loss.

Minor Aches and Pains

Seeking relief from aches and pains may have been why you chose to be introduced to massage. Perhaps you were searching for a way to feel better when your muscles began to ache. The causes of these pains can come from a wide spectrum of issues, and only a medical practitioner can really assess the causes. But minor aches and pains caused by overuse, misuse, and underuse all respond well to massage. Frequent massage encourages the blood flow to the muscles, fascia, and surrounding nerves, promoting their strength and flexibility, and helping them to thrive.

Massage relieves muscle spasms and tension, relaxing stiff muscles as circulation improves. The soreness you would normally sustain from overused muscles dissipates with frequent massage. While a person is healing from muscle strain or soreness, massage of the rest of the body is helpful in promoting good health overall.

Chronic Pain

Chronic pain is debilitating physically, mentally, emotionally, and spiritually. If you suffer from endless pain, you know that much of your life revolves around how to deal with it. Unfortunately, many people ignore the pain unless it is a major injury that must be addressed immediately. We are a society that has learned to use the "grin and bear it" option when dealing with our pain. Even worse, for many of us, our pain has been dismissed as being "all in your head."

Pain is real, whether it stems from an injury, an illness, overuse, or emotions. The pain that you feel is real. Because doctors might not know why you are in pain, you might ignore it until it becomes too big for your life, at which point you are in a chronic state of pain. Steady, unrelenting pain will wear you down. No matter how strong you are, your inner reserves will be swallowed up and diminished if you spend them all on chronic pain.

There are two classifications of pain: acute and chronic.

- **Acute pain** is sharp pain with a sudden onset. It can be caused by anything from a pinprick to a sprained ankle to a knife cut.
- **Chronic pain**, on the other hand, is slow-acting pain that begins gradually and increases in intensity. The type of feeling associated with this pain can be aching, throbbing, burning, shooting, or many other types of descriptors. The pain experience is unique to each individual. Examples of chronic pain would be the pain of arthritis or an untreated toothache. Unfortunately, some people suffer from condi-

tions such as myofascial pain syndrome (MPS) and fibromyalgia, which cause the body to be in pain for no single identifiable medically known reason (although science is trying to catch up).

> **Respecting Pain**
>
> Pain is the body's way of letting you know there is a serious problem, and it may be the signal of an internal difficulty. Always point this out to your receiver and encourage her to immediately see a doctor. Do not give a massage to someone in chronic pain until a medical professional has been consulted.

The cause of such conditions is unclear, but often involves hormone imbalances, over-receptive nerve fibers, and trigger points causing tightness and pain in the muscles. Until recently, the treatment of choice for conditions such as MPS had been to medicate, using stronger and stronger drugs to either reduce the pain or block the awareness of the pain sensation. Today a whole-body approach can be used. This approach relies on movement and relaxation techniques, including massage and trigger point therapy, to teach the sufferer how to apply self-care techniques. The specific massage routine used will depend on the nature, location, and severity of the pain.

Cardiovascular Problems

Heart disease is more prevalent today than ever before. Whether the cause is genetic or stress related, issues with the heart are generally compounded by lifestyle. Lack of exercise and foods high in bad fats and bad cholesterol weaken the muscles of the heart and overtax the blood vessels. It is now well documented that cardiovascular conditions are best treated using a combination of medical treatments and complementary therapy. Aerobic exercise is an important part of heart disease prevention; working the muscles of the body to elevate the heart rate and increase metabolism helps to keep the heart healthy. This type of exercise brings more oxygen to the muscles and prepares the body to release waste at a quicker rate.

How can massage help?

- The principles of Swedish massage enforce movements toward the heart, improving circulation and assisting the heart in its work.
- Massage improves the flow of nutrients through the body by assisting the movement of blood and lymph through the vessels, and helps to eliminate toxins.
- Each type of stroke has its own important way of helping improve circulation:
  - **Effleurage** enhances the movement of blood through the vessels close to the skin and in the muscles.
  - **Petrissage** works with the veins and arteries, stimulating the flow of blood deeper in the body.
  - **Friction** strokes work to increase the movement of the interstitial fluid as well as the circulation of lymph.

A Simple Routine to Address Cardiovascular Issues

1. Begin by lying in a comfortable position on your back. You can place a pillow under your shoulder blades to "puff out" your chest. Place your hands on your abdomen, just above and on either side of your bellybutton.
2. Notice your breathing and listen to your heartbeat. Work to slow your breath, allowing your abdomen to be fully relaxed as it rises and falls with each breath. This in turn can help to slow your heartbeat to a more relaxed rate.
3. After a minute or so, move your hands onto your sternum (breastbone). Begin slowly working your hands up and down this bone, from its bottom tip right where your ribs meet to the sternal notch, where your throat is. Repeat this ten to twelve times, all the while slowing your breath, and relaxing your muscles in the chest, neck, and face.
4. Next, extend your right arm outward and lay it on the floor. With your left hand, massage from the center of the sternum outward to the right shoulder and back again, over the pectoral muscles, or "pecs." Each time, stretch the right arm out a bit more and when you return to the sternum bone, take a starting point a bit farther down. Use massage strokes on an angle as you begin lower down the sternum, gliding upward toward the arm.
5. Repeat for the left arm.

As you become more flexible in your chest muscles, you can begin this routine lying on your back on your couch with your one arm draped off the edge while you provide the stretching strokes across the chest and pectoral muscles.

1. Next, trace a line along and just below the collarbone. Provide gliding strokes back and forth. This bone marks the uppermost edge of the pectoral muscles.
2. Complete this routine with your hands on your abdomen. Continue to breathe slowly, relaxing your neck and chest. Allow the chest and abdominal muscles to completely relax, then take a "morning stretch" ending with your arms resting over your head on the floor or surface you are lying on.

Using Massage for Cancer Patients

Cancer is an extensive subject because every system in the body can develop cancers particular to that system. But the many different diseases associated with cancer have a common denominator: the breakdown and alteration of cells, and subsequent duplication of cancerous changes to other cells. The newly mutated cells invade and erode the healthy surrounding cells, perpetuating the growth of the cancer.

Ask a Doctor First!

Although most research supports the use of massage on cancer patients, massage that stimulates the circulatory system may assist the spread of cancer. Before administering massage to a person with cancer you must get medical clearance. Moreover, it is highly recommended that you get specialized training to work with people who have cancer.

If given with the proper medical clearance, massage can be very beneficial to cancer patients for the following reasons:

- Massage helps deal with the pain related to the disease and lowers the stress level of the recipient.
- Massage helps lower blood pressure as the anxiety of the receiver decreases and muscle tension is released.
- Massage helps to support the natural immune function of the body to access its own disease-killing cells, therefore helping the body to fight the cancer.

Massaging Someone with AIDS

AIDS (acquired immune deficiency syndrome) is an infection that stems from a virus known as the human immunodeficiency virus, or HIV. The virus attacks the infection-fighting T cells on a search-and-destroy mission. As the virus spreads, it systematically seeks out and destroys the T cells, thereby destroying the body's ability to eradicate the virus. Once the immune system is disabled, HIV opens the body to a host of infections, and this condition of heightened susceptibility is the disease known as AIDS.

Know the Facts on How AIDS Is Spread

AIDS is spread through the exchange of bodily fluids, period. Not through casual contact or sweat, but through semen, breast milk, blood, and vaginal secretions. The person most at risk during a massage is an AIDS-infected receiver, not the giver, because the receiver is so susceptible to infection. The giver must be healthy so as not to compromise the already weakened state of the recipient.

Massage can be administered to someone with HIV at any time, but massage is not recommended for someone in advanced stages of AIDS. Overall, massage is a wonderful tool for providing compassionate touch, particularly to a population that is still misunderstood. Kind and loving touch will provide comfort and support, and will ease some of the worry and fear related to this disease.

Chapter 17
Trigger Point Therapy

What Is Trigger Point Therapy?

The principles of trigger point therapy are based on the concept that muscles, when chronically tight and overworked, can develop dense areas of strongly contracted fibers. These contracted areas compromise the integrity and function of the entire muscle as well as surrounding muscles and fascia. Many factors can influence the development of trigger points, such as:

- Sleep posture
- Poor nutrition
- Dehydration
- Lack of daily stretching
- Level of daily movement

Myofascial Dysfunction, Defined

Myofascial dysfunction is a commonly used diagnosis to describe pain and problems in muscles. *Myo* is Greek for "muscle" and *fascia* is all of the connective tissue that surrounds and connects every element in the human body and allows for intracellular communication and muscle function.

When harboring trigger points, muscle fibers have a local energy crisis: They don't have enough energy to run their metabolic engines and subsequently cannot relax. This creates a palpable taut band of muscle fibers that, when pressed on, can produce pain or sensation in that actual spot, or in a distant area of the body (which is called referred pain). This referred sensation happens in a predictable area, depending on which muscle it is, and it can be seen in the pain referral patterns illustrated by many researchers. For example, many people with a trigger point in their SCM (sternocleidomastiod muscle), a long stabilizing muscle in your neck, can feel pain into their head and ear; above and around the eyes; and in the forehead, like a headache. This muscle can develop trigger points and pain from sleeping on your stomach or from being in a habitually head-forward posture.

Why Doesn't My Healthcare Provider Know about Trigger Points?

Simply put, many healthcare providers don't know about trigger points. The Bone and Joint Initiative estimates that 126.6 million adults are affected by musculoskeletal pain, twice the rate of chronic heart and lung conditions. The annual U.S. cost for treatment and lost wages has been calculated to $874 billion! That is 5.7% of our entire GDP! Billions of dollars are lost each year in decreased work productivity due to muscle pain, yet trigger points are largely overlooked. Efforts to alleviate pain caused by trigger points may not bring lasting relief if the treatment focuses on the location where the pain is felt. In other words, most of our medical interventions seem to focus on the area *where* it hurts, instead of finding out and fixing *why* it hurts.

It's Fixable!

The good news is that you have the power to eliminate your own pain caused by trigger points. Through applied trigger point pressure release by a friend or trained provider, these areas can be brought back into full, pain-free function. You also have the power to press on these areas yourself through "self-massage." With these strategies, you can begin your journey into this advanced form of massage therapy. You can press using elbows, hands, fingers, and specialty tools. By applying pressure into the area of tight muscle fibers, you can begin to restore normal blood flow to the area. After a session of treatment, it is important to employ gentle movement and stretching exercises that are coordinated with relaxed breathing. With this trigger point protocol you will be on your way to healthy, strong, and pain-free muscles!

Small Trigger Points Can Cause Big Problems

A man has trouble bending down to tie his shoes because pain across his lower back prevents him from doing so. He drives an hour and a half each way to work. During the workday, he never takes a break to stand up or stretch. He slouches in front of his computer screen and does not engage in any kind of movement or exercise.

A mother of three has a chronic headache that she describes as "pain in my forehead and behind my eyes." She sleeps on her stomach with her neck twisted to the side because it's comforting to her.

A thirty-eight-year-old receptionist has tingling in her hands, thumb, and pointer finger during the day, and wakes up some nights with her hands almost numb. She thinks it is carpal tunnel syndrome.

Do any of these scenarios sound familiar to you? Do you or a loved one have unexplained pain in your muscles? If so, then it is very likely that your pain is being caused by trigger points. This chapter will explain simple changes you can make to reduce or even eliminate pain caused by trigger points, without expensive doctor visits or even pain relief medication!

Take the previous examples:

- The man with lower back pain could have trigger points in his abdominal muscles that were caused by too much sitting.
- The mom who sleeps on her stomach probably developed trigger points in her neck muscles due to her stomach-sleeping position. (Trigger points in the neck muscles are a common cause of headaches.)
- The receptionist also probably has pain from her sleeping position (which is something her doctors probably don't think to ask about). Her favorite position to sleep in is with her arms over her head or tucked around the back of her head under her pillow. She probably has trigger points in her shoulder and neck muscles caused by this awkward sleep posture. (Sleeping with arms above your head can refer tingling sensation down the arm and into the wrist, thumb, and fingers.) Making a few small changes in your habits can have a huge impact in lowering or eliminating your myofascial pain due to trigger points!

Sleep on It!

Sleep posture can greatly affect muscles. Try to sleep in the most neutral posture as possible. Side or back sleeping is best. Be sure to keep your head and neck in neutral alignment, and not bent or tucked too far forward. Avoid sleeping on the stomach.

A Brief History of Trigger Point Research

Trigger points have been recognized by many practitioners and researchers through the centuries. Austrian-born sports medicine physician Dr. Hans Kraus was using trigger point treatment concepts as early as the 1940s to get performers and athletes back into action very quickly after suffering from pain or injury. Also in the '40s, Dr. Ida P. Rolf, an early pioneer in muscular release, realized that tension in the human body caused accompanying system-wide problems. With applied held pressure she discovered that it was possible to "reshape" the connective tissue and relax deeper muscles.

Dr. Janet Travell, the first female White House physician (to President John F. Kennedy), also began researching trigger points in the early '40s. Later, she teamed up with her colleague Dr. David Simons to create the most comprehensive scientific medical books on the identification and treatment of trigger points, the two-volume set *Myofascial Pain and Dysfunction: The Trigger Point Manual; Upper Half of Body* and *Myofascial Pain and Dysfunction: The Trigger Point Manual; The Lower Extremities* (LWW, 1998, 1992).

Current Trigger Point Researchers

The growing field of myofascial pain has many contemporary researchers and leaders. Dr. Leon Chaitow, Dr. Robert Gerwin, Dr. Siegfried Mense, Dr. Helene Langevin, Dr. César Fernández-de-las-Peñas, Dr. Joanne Borg-Stein, and Jan Dommerholt DPT, just to name a few, are hard at work researching why we suffer from muscular pain and associated problems. Dr. Jay P. Shah, at the National Institutes of Health, is a lead researcher in discovering the biochemical characteristics of trigger points. He and his colleagues are helping us understand how the trigger point complex is held with the muscle fibers stuck "on," and what chemicals in there can contribute to the pain and problems that they can cause. We look forward to learning more from these leaders in this field of research.

In the late 1970s, Bonnie Prudden, a U.S. fitness pioneer and close friend of Dr. Hans Kraus, began teaching her myotherapy, a system of applied pressure and movement techniques for the elimination of pain in the muscles. Many believe that she was the first to create manual techniques from the medical textbooks developed for doctors by Drs. Travell and Simons. In 1985, the National Association of Myofascial Trigger Point Therapists (*www.myofascialtherapy.org*) was formed to serve as an educational and professional organization dedicated to teaching the public and healthcare providers about trigger point pain. They have a listing of specially trained practitioners all over the United States.

How Trigger Points Are Formed

Trigger points often form as a response to tension or strain in our muscles. We all certainly have plenty of that! Yet why don't busy children experience the same problems? If you look at joyful toddlers and children playing and moving, you'll see their muscular and skeletal system working in harmony and without unnecessary tension. As we grow and demand different things from our muscles (such as repetitive motions, frequent sitting, and so on), adaptations occur to bear the load of our efforts. Movement, in the form of play, is how children enjoy a healthy muscular system, free of trigger point pain. We could all learn something from this by trying to keep those childhood habits of play, laughter, stretching, movement, and activity in our daily lives.

> ### Prep Your Muscles for New Activities
> Trigger points can flare up when we participate in unaccustomed activities like painting an apartment or dancing the night away at a once-a-year party. Keep yourself fit and ready to use your muscles by participating in regular exercise and weight training. Then you will be ready to have fun with new activities.

Trigger points can also develop in areas of past injury and from overuse, habitual tension, or work-related (postural) tension. Do you notice that when you are stressed out that certain areas of your body seem to be under tension? Do you end up with discomfort or pain as a result? Well, as these muscles remain in the "tightened" position, the muscle cells begin to "run out of gas." That is, the energy needed to power the cells dissipates. Groups or bundles of muscle cells adapt to this dwindling energy supply by "locking" in the contracted position to conserve energy. Most of the time, when we stretch the area, perhaps by getting up from our held position to walk around, the energy crisis is over and new nutrient-filled blood can enter the area and replenish the cell's energy supply.

The Most Common Cause: Sitting for Too Long

The problem facing many adults in the workforce is sitting for extended hours working at a desk or typing on a computer. Many of us don't get up and stretch enough or don't engage in regular exercise. The tight areas with reduced energy supply can only adapt for so long. So, as we maintain these non-neutral postures (like stooping over our keyboards, slouching in our desk chairs, or bending over our cell phones), our muscles forget how to relax and a trigger point is born.

These contracted areas can limit our range of motion, reduce strength in muscles, and can send painful sensations locally or outward into what could seem like completely unrelated areas. Over time, we change the way we perform our daily tasks in fear of making this pain get worse, and the vicious cycle of trigger points begins:

1. You experience tightness
2. The tightness turns into pain
3. The pain creates reduced mobility
4. The decreased mobility causes tightness in other spots
5. That tightness turns into pain
6. That pain creates reduced mobility in another area

Today's dedicated office workers may spend up to ten hours sitting, including commute time to desk time. Consider investing in a mobile desk surface that can raise up to allow you to spend some of your day standing while still concentrating on your work.

How to Press On Trigger Points

Trigger points can be treated with a massage technique called trigger point pressure release. This pressure can be applied by a friend, a trained and certified trigger point therapist, a trained massage therapist, or other specially trained allied healthcare providers.

The client should be in a comfortable position that allows a moderate amount of stretch in the muscles, like lying on the side with one leg slightly off the table. Keep in mind that the muscles that will be worked on have been identified by the practitioner as having reduced range of motion and have been described as having some weakness or pain. Sections of the problematic muscles will have areas that will feel more dense or dysfunctional than surrounding healthy tissue. This indicates that trigger point massage needs to be applied in those areas. The process itself is very simple:

- Apply some lotion and glide your hands over the muscles that need to be treated.
- Feel for any dense segments, which are usually found in the middle of the length of the muscle.
- If you are not sure what muscle you are pressing on, you can have the receiver "press against" your resistance. This firming up allows you to feel the area while the muscles are working.
- Have the receiver exhale and relax the area while you use your fingers to feel if the muscle area actually did fully relax.
- Press firmly into the dense areas and hold for twenty to thirty seconds. Maintain steady pressure for about two or three gentle and slow breaths from the belly (diaphragm). Reduce pressure, have the recipient focus on relaxing the area, then repeat pressure in the same area. This may need to be repeated until the recipient reports lowering discomfort. Next move half an inch to another area.

Other Trigger Point Therapies

Other methods besides massage can eliminate trigger point areas in muscles. These treatments include trigger point injections, trigger point dry needling, ML830 cold laser, ultrasound, and frequency-specific microcurrent. These techniques need to be applied only by specially trained practitioners, but each can be a successful adjunct to hands-on applied pressure release.

What Am I Feeling For?

While the standard terminology uses the word *point* to describe trigger points, you are not actually going to feel any bumps, or pea-shaped lumps, or "knots," as many people describe them. You are feeling through the skin and fascia for many tens of thousands of contracted muscle cells within a muscle group that have gotten themselves stuck in the "on" position. Trying to locate the taut band that is characteristic of a trigger point area is best done by a process of trial and error: Press and feel along the length and breadth on all areas of the relevant muscles in an effort to notice any tight, banded segments that are more painful when pressed on, and that may cause a "referral" of sensation to another area. This referral sensation might locally spread out. As you press on these areas, monitor the level of sensation the receiver is experiencing with gentle questioning. "What discomfort does it cause when I press here? . . . Here? . . . Any referral of sensation to another area?" Keep the amount of discomfort at a reasonable level for the receiver.

In some areas such as the abdomen, the liopsoas muscles, are really deep, so you may only be able to feel an area of muscle that will not relax after being contracted, or an area that feels more dense than the surrounding tissue.

Where to Press and How to Find It

The main goal of trigger point therapy is to get to the root cause of the pain by following the road map given to us by Drs. Travell and Simons, who have listed all muscles that can cause or refer pain into a particular area. By following this road map, you can easily identify and eliminate the *source* of pain. A list of these muscles can be found at *www.triggerpoints.net*. On this website, follow the prompts and click on the area where you or your client have pain. All the muscles that can be causing pain in that area will be shown to you. Then use the following treatment techniques listed in this chapter.

For example, there are twelve muscles that cause pain, tingling, or sensation down the arm and into the thumb and first two fingers. Most of these muscles are not in the thumb or hand! The scalene muscle, located in the neck, is the second most probable muscle to cause pain into the thumb and index finger. In other words, if you have trigger point pain in your thumb and received medical intervention directly to your thumb, chances are likely that it would be of no use. Of the twelve muscles that can cause pain in the thumb, a muscle that is actually in the hand/thumb is number seven on the list! The rest of the muscles are high up in the shoulder and in the arm.

What to Expect from Professional Trigger Point Therapy Treatment

If you are experiencing pain that you think could be due to trigger points, you might consider finding a professional to help you before you try self-care techniques. Look for a therapist certified by the Certification Board for Myofascial Trigger Point Therapists (CB-MTPT), or for one who is listed on the National Association registry (*www.NAMTPT.org*). He or she will be familiar with the full and complete trigger point protocol.

First, you'll give a history so that the therapist can learn about you and the things you may be doing to contribute to your trigger point pain or myofascial dysfunction. These things are called perpetuating factors.

Next, the therapist will assess the ability of the muscles to stretch. The therapist will then use the Travell and Simons's books to determine which muscles to treat using trigger point pressure release and advanced massage techniques. This is a dynamic and interactive protocol. You will be in communication with the therapist for the entire session as you work to regain full muscle function. You will then be given self-care homework—techniques like compression and stretching—to keep the muscles fully functioning.

Self-Applied Trigger Point Techniques

While it is a good idea to seek treatment from a trained professional, we are all capable of applying trigger point pressure release on our tight and contracted muscle segments. Just like brushing our teeth, we all should exercise good muscle hygiene by using massage techniques to keep our fascia and muscles in tip-top shape.

Here are some general tips for self-applied trigger point pressure release:

- Warm up the area with five minutes of gentle cardio exercise, a warm compress, or a warm shower.
- It is usually best to apply pressure with a tool using only gravity or body weight. (Commonly used tools for self-applied trigger point work are noted later in this chapter.)

- Remain relaxed and don't "use" the muscle that is being pressed on; it will hurt more. Use a coordinated exhale along with mindful "letting go" of muscle tension.
- Monitor discomfort and only achieve levels of "hurts so good." This is an individual rating scale. Use a scale of one to ten, with ten being the worst pain you've ever felt, and stay within the five to six range.
- Keep the area being treated in a supported and stretched position.
- Focus on the exhale phase of breathing and don't overbreathe in a shallow way from the chest. Breathing and relaxation go hand in hand. When applying self-compression, focus on noticing if you are holding your breath or your muscles are tight. If you notice that you are doing either or both of these things, gently squeeze your muscles while you breathe in from your lower belly, and then coordinate an exhale with a complete release of the created tension.
- Make a mental note of any areas that were more tender or that you pressed on and it replicated some of your trigger point pain. Return and press on these areas; they are important.

> Simple changes in your life can have a profound impact on your muscular health. Without assessing for and eliminating these things, your pain may not fully go away, or may keep coming back over time. Sleep posture should be as close to a neutral posture as possible. Proper seated posture at work could include the use of an adjustable chair. Create a work station in which you are relaxed and able to sit comfortably while using the phone, keyboard, mouse, files, and so forth.

How Much Is Enough?

Some people find it necessary to press really hard on their trigger point areas in order to "feel" that they are getting full relief into the area. The general rule of thumb is to press only until the "hurts so good" point is reached. Trigger point pressure should not be painful, per se; rather, it should feel therapeutically beneficial and helpful. The good thing about self-applied pressure is that you are always in complete control of how much or how little pressure is used in any area.

To start out, hold pressure on important areas for approximately two or three gentle slow breaths. Then you can move your compression to another area a half inch away from that spot. Repeat this process, and make special note of the places that were exquisitely tender. Then go back to those places and begin the whole process again.

Commonly Used Tools

You'll need a few inexpensive tools in order to use the self-care techniques described in this chapter. They're readily available at massage supply stores or online. Here are some top choices:

- Backnobber Massager (*www.triggerpointproducts.com*): An S-shaped tool used for deep massage of the muscles of the upper or lower back or neck.
- Jacknobber Massager (*www.triggerpointproducts.com*): A small knobbed tool to help apply precise pressure.
- Stretch Out Strap (*www.optp.com/Stretch-Out-Straps*): Woven straps that allow you to stretch safely and effectively without a partner.
- Tiger Tail (*www.tigertailusa.com*): A foam-covered massage stick that delivers even pressure on large muscles.
- FitBall (*www.fitball.com*): Trigger point compression ball that is available in several sizes.
- Curve Ball (*www.tigertailusa.com*): A curved foam massage surface with a grippy base that allows for deep muscle pressure without the movement of a ball.
- Tiger Ball (*www.tigertailusa.com*): A 2.6-inch silicone ball able to slide along the length of a reinforced rope allowing access to hard-to-reach places and good control of trigger point compression.

Trigger Point Therapy for Specific Areas of Pain

The following sections will show you how to address specific muscles that could be causing local or referred pain. Again, refer to *www.triggerpoints.net* to determine which muscle you might need to work on based on where you have your pain. Click on your area of pain, and the list of muscles that need to be worked on will pop up.

Head and Headaches on the Front of the Face

A headache that seems to start on the side of the neck and move into the areas of the eyebrows, jaw, or cheeks is a very common referral pattern from the trigger points in the upper trapezius muscle.

Tool Used and Where: Backnobber on Upper Trapezius

To best self-treat this muscle, use the Original Backnobber Massager self-care tool. Apply pressure using the knob at the end of the smaller curve of the Backnobber.

1. Start seated on a chair, comfortably supported.
2. Reach the smaller curved end of the Backnobber until it is placed almost right on "top" of the shoulder. With the opposite hand, press into the uppermost curve of the tool so the pressure goes downward directly into the upper shoulder muscles and portions of the longer neck muscles.
3. Next, add some element of stretch as shown in Figure 38: Lean your body over the opposite of the side being treated, and allow your head and neck to side bend. Press on the tool with less power because the muscles are in a stretched position and may be more sensitive.

Forehead, Eyebrow, or Ear

When experiencing pain in the forehead or eyebrow, or fullness or ringing in the ear, trigger points in the sternocleidomastoid muscles (SCM) along the sides of your neck may be a culprit.

Technique Used and Where: Pincer Technique on the SCM

To find this muscle, gently place your fingers at the notch just between your collarbones. Move a half inch to the right side, tilt your head to the right side, and rotate your chin to the left. You may feel the SCM muscle stick out a little. (See Figure 39.)

1. Using pincer pressure, begin at this area, gripping the SCM muscle between your middle and pointer finger and thumb. The pincer technique is a fancy way of describing your fingers working like a "pincer" or claw of a crab gently on muscle

and fascia. Be sure you have the muscle between your pincer grasp and not just the skin of the neck. Continue to work upward almost all the way up to the ear.

2. After compression is complete, gently stretch the area by rotating your head to look "behind you." Gently encourage further stretching by using the opposite hand to press the head further into the rotation as you fully relax the neck muscles.

Neck and Headaches in the Back of the Head

Trigger points in the deep, uppermost neck muscles can cause headaches that wrap around the head or are into the back of the head or hurt into the eye.

Tool Used and Where: Backnobber on the Suboccipital Muscles

1. While seated, place the Backnobber's smaller curved end on the neck muscles just below the base of your skull on the right side. Be sure not to press directly into the notch at the center of your neck.
2. Press your right hand upward on the bottom curve of the Backnobber while your left hand grasps the topmost part of the other curve and pulls downward on the tool.
3. Tilt your head downward and look to your left armpit, then look to your right armpit. (See Figure 40.)
4. To stretch afterward, move the head slowly in all directions, as if touching the hours on a clock. Come back to a neutral or center position before moving on.

Stiff Neck

The levator scapulae muscle is also known as "the stiff neck muscle." Trigger points in this muscle can cause discomfort into the area where the neck meets the upper back and shoulder and can prevent us from twisting the neck or from bending the neck to the side.

Tool Used and Where: Backnobber Just Next to the Shoulder Blade

1. To treat this muscle, use a Backnobber to press into the upper right back at the upper edge of the shoulder blade (as shown in Figure 41).

2. To add stretch, turn the head to the left, bend the neck to look into the left armpit, and exhale as you press.
3. To stretch afterward, bring your right arm behind you as if you are reaching for your left back pocket. Grasp your right wrist and press down with your left hand while you bend your neck to the left and look to the left armpit.

Shoulder

Pain in the front of the shoulder can make us think we have "injured" our rotator cuff. Often, this *front* of shoulder pain is actually referred from a muscle in the *back*; the infraspinatus muscle.

Tool Used and Where: Tennis Ball (or Tiger Ball) on Infraspinatus Muscle

1. To treat this muscle, stand next to a wall with your feet slightly in a lunge about 6–12 inches from the wall. Holding on to the rope, hang the Tiger Ball over your shoulder until it comes in contact with your left shoulder blade bone.
2. Gently apply a small amount of your body weight onto the ball as it presses against the wall and into the muscles. Cross your left arm in front of your chest to stretch the infra and gently lean weight onto the Tiger Ball (as shown in Figure 42).
3. Move around on the ball and look for any more tender areas. Repeat the compression. If you feel a discomfort in the front of your shoulder or down your arm, you have found trigger points in your infraspinatus muscle!

Lower Back Pain ("My Back Went Out!")

Pain in the lower and mid-back could actually be referred pain from trigger points in muscles in the abdomen.

Tool Used and Where: FitBall on the Psoas and Rectus Abdominis Muscles

1. Stage 1: Place a 5- or 7-inch FitBall body therapy ball at your bellybutton or below, then lean against a wall, pressing into the ball.

2. Stage 2: To take it to the next level, lie on your side on the floor. Bring the ball toward your mid-belly and gently roll onto the ball and "melt" into the ball as you relax your abdominal muscles and fascia.

3. Stage 3: The same concept applies for the final and advanced technique (as shown in Figure 43). Lie on your stomach and place the FitBall at your pubic bone, resting your body on your elbows. With this method, you have the ability to control the amount of weight that goes onto the ball by graduating the way you rest your body onto the ball. If needed, you can use a pillow under the upper chest to relieve some weight that goes onto the ball.

Lower Back Pain Caused by Sitting in Poor Posture

Another source of pain in the lower to mid-back can be trigger points in the spinal erector muscles. These muscles can become chronically weak and tight due to poor sitting and standing posture, poor ergonomics, or underuse.

Tool Used and Where: Backnobber on Torso

1. To use the Backnobber on the spinal erector muscles, bring the larger curved end of the tool around your torso and place it against the paraspinal muscles on the left side. (If you are large of stature, keep the knobble on the right side muscles.) See Figure 44. This company also makes a larger version called the "Big Bend" for persons of larger or heavier stature.

2. To add stretch, rotate and bend your torso forward at the waist while you gently apply compression. See Figure 45. Breathe, relax, and release pressure on the tool as you come upright.

Buttocks Pain

Pain in the buttocks can be very challenging especially when walking or sitting for any length of time. Trigger points in the gluteus medius and minimus can cause pain that makes walking difficult and can cause tension in the hip.

Tool Used and Where: FitBall on the Glutes

As a rule of thumb, use the least amount of pressure when you begin self-care.

1. Stage 1: You may prefer to compress your glute muscles by pressing a ball against a wall while standing.
2. Stage 2: Then you can graduate to using the ball on a couch or bed.
3. Stage 3: Finally, try the hard surface of the floor. Begin by placing the ball under your glute muscles on the left side (as shown in Figure 46). Roll the ball over the full area of your buttocks and hip. Then begin a slow and systematic treatment of specific areas holding for two or three breaths. If you do not feel discomfort, move an inch to another area. Return to areas that were particularly painful, or that caused you to feel relief or pain in another area. As always, you have the power to decide how much pressure to apply by leaning your body onto or off of the tool.

Hip Pain

If you feel pain or discomfort along the side edge of your hip/buttocks area, you may have trigger points in your tensor fasciae latae (TFL) muscle, a hip stabilizer. Sometimes this pain is mistaken for bursitis of the hip.

Tool Used and Where: Jacknobber on the Hip

1. To use the Jacknobber, place it against the wall. Cross the leg closest to the wall behind the other leg, and then gently lean the front/side edge of your hip/thigh into the knobble end of the tool, as shown in Figure 47.
2. If you don't feel stable doing this while standing, consider the techniques previously described for using the 5" FitBall while on the floor instead.

Thigh or Knee Pain

Your quadriceps muscles, known as "quads," are strong muscles that move your knee and flex your hip. The uppermost thigh is the area that most likely harbors trigger points that can refer pain all the way down the thigh and into the front of the knee. However, it is important to massage the entire length of these muscles.

Tool Used and Where: Tiger Tail on the Thigh

1. In a comfortable seated position, bend the knee by placing one foot behind you. Be sure not to have a bend in the top of the thigh; keep that area extended.
2. Hold firmly on both sides of the Tiger Tail and press the tool into the uppermost part of the thigh muscles, just below your hip pointer or iliac crest, as shown in Figure 48.
3. Roll the Tiger Tail along the length of the thigh from the top to the bottom, massaging and lengthening the fibers of these strong and hardworking muscles.

"Buckling Knee" Pain

Trigger points in the lowermost segment of the thigh muscle (vastus medialis) can refer pain just above and into the knee and can cause the knee to feel unstable, weak, or to actually give out for no reason.

Tool Used and Where: Curve Ball with Stretch Strap on the Thigh

1. Lie facedown with your mid to lowermost thigh on top of the Curve Ball. Wrap a stretch strap (or a dog leash or rope strap) around your foot.
2. Grasp a part of the strap and gently bring your foot toward your buttocks, stretching the thigh muscles, as shown in Figure 49.
3. Hold steady for two or three slow relaxing breaths, then move your body upward about an inch or two, placing it back down on the tool.
4. Work your way down the remaining length of the quad muscles to just above the knee.

Heel and Achilles Pain

Trigger points in the soleus (calf muscle) can cause referred pain into the heel and Achilles tendon area. These trigger points can also cause weakness in your walking stride, especially when pushing off your toes.

Tool Used and Where: Stretch Out Strap and Jacknobber on Calf

1. When compressing the soleus muscle you should find a comfortable spot on the floor and place your back to a wall. Run your hands over the backs of your calves and feel for any spots that are painful or harder or denser than the surrounding tissue. You will most likely be feeling the gastrocnemius muscle, as this muscle lies on top of the soleus, but compression in this area will still be beneficial to the soleus. Focus on the lower two-thirds of the calf.

2. Place the loop of a Stretch Out Strap (or a dog leash or rope strap) around the ball of your foot.

3. Starting at the lower one-third of the calf, place the Jacknobber tool under your calf while making sure your toes are pointing toward the ceiling. Once the Jacknobber tool is under your calf, pull on the strap, making the back of your calf taut and in a stretched position. (See Figure 50.)

4. Let your leg rest on top of the knobby part of the Jacknobber tool for two or three breaths, and then move the tool in 1-inch intervals. You can also hold the Jacknobber in your hand and apply pressure to the calf that way.

Chapter 18

Specialized Massage and Bodywork Techniques

The Foundations of Eastern Medicine

The different forms of massage and bodywork—the techniques and the benefits unique to each one—are rooted in the cultures that developed them. The techniques we use today come from those developed in China, Japan, Thailand, India, and Sweden, to name just a few. Whenever you give a massage, you use a combination of techniques that are connected to a variety of bodywork systems, many of them ancient.

Traditional Eastern medical principles are based on the concept of the uninterrupted flow of life force through hundreds of meridians and acupressure points in the body.

The Life Force

The life force, or vital force, is the energy that is present in you and that exists all around you. Everything consists of energy; only the packaging is different. Think of it as something similar to the Force that Luke Skywalker learns about from his master Yoda in the Star Wars movie series. The free flow of this energy insures harmonious functioning of the body's organ systems, emotions, and spirit. On the other hand, blocked energy can disrupt health and the feeling of well-being. Disorders of energy flow can disrupt your health and the feeling of well-being.

What the Life Force Is Called in Different Cultures

Qi, or *ch'i*, is the Chinese name for your vital life force, the energy of the universe that flows through you and all matter, and the thread that connects us all. In Japanese culture it is known as *ki*, in India it is *prana*, and in Tibet it is *lung* (or *rlung*).

Meridians

Energy flows through the body along an uninterrupted path of interconnected channels called meridians. The meridians are the pathways through which the vital life force flows. Traditional Chinese medicine makes use of these channels through acupressure and acupuncture to balance the energy flow within the body, stimulating the healer within and allowing the body to heal itself.

There are twelve main meridians and eight meridians known as extraordinary vessels.

The main meridians run on either side of the body, six beginning or ending in the hands and six beginning or ending in the feet. The meridians allow for the free flow of energy, blood, and fluids in the body, facilitating health The vessels form a conduction system that provides fuel for the organs and feeds the body at large. The twelve main meridians are as follows:

1. Lung
2. Large intestine
3. Stomach
4. Spleen/pancreas
5. Heart
6. Small intestine
7. Bladder
8. Kidney
9. Gall bladder
10. Pericardium
11. Liver
12. Triple burner

The energetic functions of the main meridians are the same as the functions of the organs with which connect; treat the points along a meridian and you treat the organ related to that energy line. In massage, acupressure applied by the fingers works specific points on meridian pathways, either concentrating on one point or moving along the entire meridian line, depending on the massage.

Meridians circulate qi, just as blood flows through arteries and veins, as lymph flows through lymph vessels, and as nerve signals follow a pathway. All of these circuits travel continuously throughout the entire body through every system, from one organ to another, through every part of the body to ensure balance.

Yin and Yang

The concept of yin and yang is central to traditional Chinese medicine. The qualities of yin and yang are complementary and mutually dependent; they represent the duality of nature. Yin represents the female force, and yang represents the male force. Yin is the feminine passive principle in nature that in Chinese cosmology is exhibited in darkness, cold, or wetness; yang is the masculine active principle in nature that is exhibited in light, heat, or dryness. Together, yin and yang combine to produce all that comes to be. Because you are part of the universe, you have these opposing, yet balancing, forces within you. In the body, the internal regions are yin and the external regions are yang. For example, the muscles and bones are yin and the skin is yang. Looking from a physiological standpoint, yin stores the energy and yang performs the activities. The goal of Eastern treatment is to balance yin and yang by opening the flow of energy along the meridian channels and restoring harmony.

The Five Elements

According to Chinese thinking, five elements make up the world: metal, water, wood, fire, and earth. These are the natural forces essential for life. Although termed "elements," these categories deal with the energy forces that are the conditions of being. You are comprised of these five elements, because you are part of nature. Imagine a wheel, a continuum of energy that has no beginning and no end. The elements are such entities that one element flows along the circle producing another element, and so on. The relationship between these elements within your body represents the quality of your health.

Traditional Chinese Medicine

Traditional Chinese medicine (TCM) consists of four methods of treatment: acupuncture, herbs/diet, massage (tui na), and meditation (qi gong). Backed by thousands of years of study and application, the principles of this system are used to maintain good health and prevent disease. TCM focuses on the cause of the discomfort rather than the symptoms.

The classic Chinese medical book *The Yellow Emperor's Classic of Internal Medicine* (University of California Press, 2002), or *Neijing Suwen*, is believed to have been compiled in the early Han dynasty (206 B.C. to A.D. 220) and documents the whole spectrum of Chinese medical arts. Today, traditional Chinese medicine and modern Western techniques are used together in China, and the value of this integration is becoming appreciated and accepted in the West as well.

Acupressure

Acupressure is applied pressure through finger, thumb, and hand movements to specific points on the energy meridians. This ancient Chinese method of healing is the model for many other pressure-point therapies, such as shiatsu and tui na. Pressing the meridian points on the patient's body, from the fingertips to the feet and along the lines between the meridians, sends messages to the brain along the meridians. A fully clothed patient lies on a mat as the practitioner presses the points along the energy meridians. This gentle, noninvasive work relieves stress, relaxes the body and the mind, improves blood circulation, relieves muscle aches and pains, aids in the removal of toxins, and encourages whole-body health. Acupressure deals with the patient as a whole—every point connects to every other point within the body, and all these points connect to the mind and spirit as well. Acupressure works to restore homeostasis; as the body is balanced, harmony returns. Shiatsu is gentle and generally clothed. Tui na is very diverse, and can be quite vigorous. Usually the patient is not fully clothed.

Tui Na

The bodywork system of tui na uses a variety of techniques from traditional Chinese medicine, including massage, joint mobilization, acupressure, and moxibustion (the burning of dried mugwort for healing). Tui na uses a combination of these techniques in a variety of ways, depending upon the need of the patient. The flow of energy, ch'i, is considered and the meridians are used to restore balance. Tui na is often used in conjunction with foods and exercise to promote true healing. A tui na practitioner diagnoses the recipient by feeling his pulse. Today doctors in China study tui na along with acupuncture and herbs.

The Japanese System

The Japanese method of healing uses the basic precepts of yin and yang, the five elements, and meridians. The balance of ki, the life-force energy, is elemental to the work of shiatsu, the Japanese system of finger pressure. In shiatsu, pressure is applied to tsubo points, located along the meridians. The response of the nervous system is a total body/mind reaction. Traditional Japanese medicine also involves Kampo treatment, the medical use of herbs indigenous to Japan.

Shiatsu

Shiatsu is the Japanese word for finger pressure. Shiatsu uses finger and hand pressure, combined with gentle manual manipulation of the body, to work with the life force, ki, to promote healing. Shiatsu works toward whole health, and its goal is to bring the opposite poles (yin and yang) into balance while restoring the flow of ki. The process involves the pressing of tsubo points along the meridians, which are the energy lines that access every organ and body part. This form of touch appears simple in action, but requires great skill to enlist the vital life force to come into balance. Every point that receives pressure calls out for harmony throughout the body, mind, and spirit. Regular sessions of shiatsu teach the body to recognize harmony as the desired state of being.

Fully clothed, the receiver sits and then lies on a mat or cushion while the giver presses points along the energy lines. The giver also stretches and rotates certain areas of the receiver's body as part of the routine. The release of toxins, tension, and energy blocks leaves the receiver of shiatsu feeling relaxed and energized when the session is over.

The Tsubo Point

Tsubo is the exact point on a meridian where shiatsu is applied. When pressure is applied to the tsubo point, underlying congestion is dissipated and harmony is restored through improvement the flow of ki, the vital force. Proper application of pressure brings internal and external balance.

Kampo

The Kampo system of herbalism, which has been time-tested over more than a thousand years, uses particular herbs to treat specific symptoms. The particular herbs deal with the individual's response to the illness (the symptoms), not the cause or cure of the illness itself. Kampo deals with a person's *sho*, which is the person's response to emotional, physical, mental, spiritual, and social conditions. To bring a person's ki back into harmony, his sho must be in balance.

Herbs are administered in combination or singly, depending upon the state of the client's sho. There are hundreds of formulas to match every condition of sho that may surface. Generally, Kampo formulas have no serious side effects, making a Kampo treatment seem more desirable than many drugs. The herbs used in this system have many active ingredients, allowing for better use of the primary ingredient while leaving very little chance of toxic reaction. Some Kampo practitioners provide a shiatsu treatment along with herbal treatment; others will refer the receiver to a qualified shiatsu practitioner.

Thai Massage

Traditional massage from Thailand dates back 2,500 years. The "Father Doctor" Jivaka Kumar Bhaccha, an Indian devotee of Buddha, is credited with the development of Thai massage. In early times, Thai massage was used to treat many different ailments such as liver and respiratory disorders and muscle weakness. Today, this massage is beneficial in treating soft-tissue and muscle soreness as well as helping to restore mobility. Thai massage also helps to reduce stress and restore balance. Recipients of this massage feel renewed and strong with increased energy.

The recipient is fully clothed for a Thai massage session, except shoes and socks. Thai massage is provided to the receiver on a mat while the giver moves around the mat, gently repositioning the receiver into stretches. The giver then uses thumbs, palms, or even feet to press certain points along the energy lines of the body. The application of sustained pressure on specific points along the meridian lines opens up the energy channels. The practitioner continues from the points to a series of stretches that support the release of blockages and keep the energy flowing. Recipients of this massage feel renewed and strong with increased energy. This ancient tradition has been brought into the modern era by some specially trained practitioners who also use Thai massage in a clinical setting to eliminate trigger points, restore range of motion, and get rid of pain.

Ayurvedic Tradition

Ayurveda, translated as "the science of life," means to know how to live in health. The Ayurvedic tradition for perfect health includes the concepts of meditation, yoga, massage, nutrition, and herbal medicine. The principles of Ayurvedic wisdom come from 5,000 years of work and study in this ancient Indian tradition. The process involves body-mind education and healing by influencing the nervous system. Its purpose is to reunite the individual self with the higher self, or pure conscious self.

Balancing *prana*, the universal life force, brings inner harmony and well-being. Ayurvedic treatment works on the pranic level first, then moves into the physical. As the energy of the prana is worked, the nervous system begins the healing process, sending a message to the physical, which sends a corrected message to the brain.

Ayurvedic thinking supports positive wellness, with no room for negative thoughts, feelings, or behaviors. The freedom to be whole and healthy is within all of us, and it is up to each of us to take the steps to find freedom from pain, disease, discomfort, and fear. We all have the ability within us to be free from all limitations. All is possible. The practices of yoga, meditation, and guided visualization are essential to Ayurvedic thought. The use of herbs externally and internally is also an essential part of the Ayurvedic tradition, as is eating simple yet elegant foods, which feed the body as well as the soul.

Yoga

Yoga is the ageless system of healing that is integral to the Ayurvedic tradition. Yoga teaches us to be centered and to focus on the moment. Yoga teaches you how to breathe correctly, and how to use your breath to get the most from your body.

Yoga is a way of life. Once you begin to consciously and responsibly practice yoga, your life will change for the better. As you breathe properly and understand the movement of your body, you begin to embrace the divine within. You recognize, through facing your own weakness, that we are truly all the same.

Ayurvedic Massage

The concept of Ayurvedic medicine comes through in the Ayurvedic system of massage. Ayurveda means the science of life, and its purpose is to provide a lifestyle that will provide whole health through understanding how the mind influences the body. This principle promotes self-awareness of body and mind. Balance is the recipe.

Balance of body, mind, and spirit is promoted through the basic concepts of right diet, thought, exercise, intention, giving, and compassion. Massage is an important part of healthcare with this system. A self-massage before you bathe in the morning is recommended to help rid the body of toxins and stimulate the system.

Ayurvedic massage is a tool to use every day, with oil or without. Massage your head as though you were giving yourself a shampoo, and then use long, gliding strokes down your body, over your chest, as much of your back as you can reach, and finally your arms and legs. Rub your feet between your hands and press on your toes. This is a wonderful way to begin your day, and even better if you do some yoga stretches before the massage.

Other Ancient Traditions

The art of healing touch has been passed down from generation to generation by a variety of different cultures. Several of these traditions remain today, proving just how beneficial these massage techniques can be.

Reflexology

Reflexology is an ancient form of healing touch that is physical and energetic. It classically exemplifies the greater world of bodywork. More than a foot rub but not a massage, this work uses thumbs and fingers to apply pressure to specific points on the feet, hands, and ears that in turn represent the greater body. Working these points, zones, and meridians on the feet affects the whole body. When you work on the sole, you touch the soul.

Each foot has more than 7,000 nerve pathways that flow through the body to the brain, and then from the brain to other parts of the body. Through the use of reflexology the giver can release stress, promote circulation, and help remove toxins. At the same time, the receiver relaxes on such a deep level that when the treatment is finished, the receiver feels trouble-free. Reflexology continues to work long after the touch has ended, helping to keep the receiver stress-free.

Reiki

Reiki is energy healing work. Dr. Mikao Usui, a Buddhist monk and spiritual teacher who studied and traveled the world searching for powerful healing tools, reintroduced this ancient form of touch. This healing work is applied following a systematic pattern that connects with the chakras. After a program of study, the practitioner may either place her hands directly on the receiver or lift her hands up into the aura.

Reiki calms the nerves, reduces stress, and promotes overall relaxation. It helps to diminish pain, and restores energy and vitality to the receiver. Reiki is so simple that a child can practice this loving form of healing, yet Reiki is so powerful it can seem miraculous. Documented cases show Reiki combined with conventional medicine can relieve many symptoms and assist in the healing process. Reiki connects you with your divine energy, allowing you to give unconditionally, with kindness and compassion.

Lomilomi

Lomilomi is a traditional form of Hawaiian healthcare, originally known only by the indigenous families of Hawaii. It is a native form of medical massage used to work on injuries and muscle tension to relieve muscle spasms, increase flexibility, improve circulation and respiration, stimulate the central nervous system, and help with digestion. The concept of this healing technique is to touch upon the ability of the receiver to heal herself. Medical practitioners in Hawaii may refer a client to a lomilomi practitioner. This integrative and complementary treatment is recognized as being helpful in the treatment and recovery of illness and injury and, as such, is covered by healthcare insurance.

The Swedish Method of Massage

This method is the mainframe of modern-day massage. The Swedish system of massage takes into account anatomy, physiology, and the way the body's functions and systems respond to particular manipulations and strokes. Swedish massage utilizes the movements that come naturally to humans—glides, kneads, pinches, twists, presses, taps, pulls, shakes, and stretches—to work on the soft tissue and underlying muscles, releasing toxic waste and promoting circulation. Swedish massage is the number-one choice for stress reduction. Athletes want this form of massage because it stimulates their muscles before an event and releases the knots and tension after an event.

Swedish massage can be soft and gentle, deep and firm, and stimulating, all at one session. This type of massage is very effective for chronic pain, because the strokes can be used to reach deep into the tissue, releasing adhesions while teaching the muscles new memories for how to function properly. The main physiological effects of Swedish massage are the relaxation and stimulation it provides to the muscles, the circulatory system, and the endocrine system.

Swedish massage improves skin tone because improved circulation of the blood increases the oxygen supply that feeds the skin. The nervous system benefits also, whether slowing down or speeding up, depending upon the particular need of the body being massaged. Swedish massage is beneficial in almost all instances, although some conditions require clearance from a medical practitioner.

Deep-Tissue Massage

Deep-tissue massage is the application of a variety of strokes that affect the deep tissues and fascia of the body. This massage is directed toward the supportive and dynamic matrix of fascia—the collagen system covering, surrounding, and interpenetrating the entire muscular system—to keep the soft tissue system moving freely. Deep-tissue massage techniques work to release the physical tension and restrictions in the muscle tissue, encouraging mobility and freedom from pain. These physiological procedures are often combined with psychological release brought about by the deep bodywork as the pressure opens old restrictions. The work of deep-tissue massage actually changes the physical structure of the body, aligning the core of the body both physically and emotionally. The idea is to realign the structure of the body by improving posture and releasing restrictions in the muscles. The spine and muscles hold the memories of proper body function as well as past trauma, so to fix the spine and the structures that support it means fixing the whole body.

The Trager Technique

The Trager technique is a form of deep structural integration developed by Dr. Milton Trager. The Trager technique teaches the receiver to relax as mobility is regained. There are two parts to this method:

1. The first is a series of rhythmic stretching and rocking movements administered by the giver, who shakes the parts of the receiver's body that are constricted, such as tight muscles and painful joints. The point of this movement is to produce a state of deep relaxation.
2. Second, the receiver learns a number of movements to practice at home. These movements support the relaxation and mobility that the giver has introduced.

Rolfing

Rolfing is a form of deep-tissue massage named for its developer, Dr. Ida Rolf. Rolfing helps to align the spine and body so that the organs will function properly. Dr. Rolf discovered that poor posture from childhood creates a misalignment that causes long-term problems such as poor body structure, poor muscle tone, and interference with the functions of the internal organs. Rolfing reshapes the body's posture and realigns the muscles and connective tissue. This deep work is performed with fingers, knuckles, closed fist, or elbow.

A Lifetime of Balance

Bodywork and massage help to keep us in balance. The role of massage and bodywork and their many variations continues to grow in acceptance. As you learn about and start to practice various techniques, see if you can feel the differences. Some are subtle and some are obvious. Let your hands and fingers continue to guide you on this limitless journey of touch.

Appendix A: Glossary

abdomen:
The structure in the center of the body that holds the visceral organs; the center of the life-force energy, or qi.

acupressure:
A form of traditional Chinese medicine in which fingers are used to press into the energy points on the meridians to promote healing by releasing congestion and allowing the life force, or qi, to flow clearly.

acupuncture:
A traditional Chinese medicine practice that uses needles inserted into energy points along the meridians to promote wellness; the points are energetically connected to the organs of the body and the needles free congestion to bring balance and harmony.

adrenal glands:
The hormone-producing glands that sit on top of the kidneys.

adrenaline:
The main fight-or-flight hormone produced by the adrenal gland.

anatomy:
The study of the structure of the body.

anatripsis:
The art of rubbing the skin up toward the heart using the flow of the circulatory system to rid the body of waste; discovered by Hippocrates.

anmo:
The original form of massage healing used in ancient China.

aromatherapy:
A therapeutic treatment using medicinal-quality essential oils.

Ayurveda:
An ancient Indian form of medicine that combines yoga, meditation, massage, and herbal medicine to promote a healing lifestyle.

baths:
Used today to promote healing and relaxation with water; originated in ancient times.

bodywork:
Any form of touch that uses techniques to bring about change and healing; not necessarily massage.

chair massage:
A seated massage with the person fully dressed; can be performed anywhere and can be as short as ten minutes.

chakras:
Energy points within the body that keep a sense of balance through connections with the endocrine and central nervous systems.

chiropractor:
A doctor of natural medicine who treats the spine to heal the body.

connective tissue:
Tissue that supports and binds together other tissues. It includes such fibrous tissue as tendons, ligaments, and cartilage; and it provides support and protection while holding everything in the body together.

connective tissue massage:
Deep massage that helps rid the body of toxins in the muscles.

deep-tissue massage:
Swedish massage as it is used with more applied pressure to work deep into the fascia to free restrictions in muscle tissue.

drape:
A form of covering used during massage to allow the receiver to feel safe and secure.

effleurage:
A Swedish massage term used to describe long, gliding strokes; this stroke is a mainstay of massage therapy.

endocrine system:
The system that produces all the hormones of the body.

energy work:
A type of bodywork that works with the vital life force of the body (qi) to release congestion and promote balance.

essential oils:
Natural oils derived from plants and distilled with steam to produce the essence of the plant; they can be used for medicinal, therapeutic, or cosmetic purposes.

fascia:
The three-dimensional fibrous tissue matrix that connects to and communicates with the entire muscular system and the whole human body.

fight-or-flight response:
Our instinctual response to an emergency that tells us to fight off the enemy or flee; produces increased blood pressure, heart and respiratory rates, and skeletal muscle blood flow, all of which is not useful in most present-day stressful situations.

friction:
A massage stroke that moves the skin over the muscle, releasing tension and breaking up adhesions.

gymnasium:
An institution of ancient Greece where athletics, massage, and debate took place; the modern-day version is the spa.

homeostasis:
The state of equilibrium; the preferred state of the body.

hydrotherapy:
Any water therapy; a direct descendant from the Greek gymnasium.

interstitial fluid:
The fluid in between the cells and blood vessels.

ischemia:
A condition where the blood flow to the muscles is constricted, causing pain.

ki:
The Japanese word for the vital life-force energy.

kneading:
A technique in Swedish massage, also known as petrissage, that is performed as though the massage therapist is kneading dough.

ligament:
A tough fibrous band of connective tissue that connects bone to bone, or keeps an organ in place.

lymph:
Fluid that helps feed the cells. It plays a key role in fighting infection by taking toxins away from the body.

lymph drainage:
A process that helps the lymph system to function, reducing swelling and releasing toxins.

massage:
The manual manipulation of the soft tissues of the body.

meridians:
The life-force energy channels that run through the body; there are twelve main meridians and six vessels used in acupuncture, acupressure, and many other forms of bodywork.

metabolism:
The internal process within the body that transforms food to energy.

muscle fatigue:
The condition of a muscle when it has worked so hard that it does not respond when contracted.

muscle spasm:
The involuntary contraction of a muscle or a number of muscles; can result from abnormal levels of electrolytes or minerals in the body

nervous system:
The system comprising the brain and spinal cord, nerves, and ganglia that receives and interprets stimuli and transmits impulses throughout the body tissue.

pain:
The sensation a body creates to let the individual know if something is wrong with the function of the body; the body's alarm system.

palpation:
The examination of the body by feeling with hands and fingers, such as in massage.

petrissage:
The kneading technique used in massage.

physiology:
The study of the functions of the body.

prana:
The Sanskrit word for the vital life-force energy.

pressure points:
Specific points that run along the meridians and that are connected to particular organs; used in forms of therapy such as acupuncture and acupressure.

qi:
A term used in Chinese healing that represents the vital life-force energy in the body.

referred pain:
Pain or sensation that can be replicated when pressing on a trigger point; often felt at a distance away from where one is pressing.

reflexology:
A system of bodywork using points in the feet, hands, and ears to treat the entire body; brings deep relaxation and physical relief from illness.

Reiki
A system of energy work in which the giver works with the receiver's energy field, known as the aura; provides a deep sense of well-being and promotes healing.

shiatsu:
An ancient traditional Japanese finger-pressure treatment; adapted from the Chinese anmo and tui na techniques.

sports massage:
A special massage for athletes using mostly Swedish techniques; given before an event to stimulate, after the event for relaxation, and during training to maintain muscle fitness.

stress:
The stimulus that makes the body respond with the production of adrenaline; if the stimulus is not dispelled, the body continuously reacts with a fight-or-flight response.

Swedish massage:
The mainframe of modern-day massage; a system of massage that uses movements known as effleurage, petrissage, and tapotement to work on the soft tissue and underlying muscles to help release toxic waste and promote circulation.

tapotement:
The tapping, percussive strokes in Swedish massage.

tendon:
Dense fibrous connective tissue that unites a muscle with a bone.

Thai massage:
An ancient form of healing that balances the qi, using pressure on the healing points and passive stretching.

trigger point:
A highly dense and hyperirritable grouping of thousands of muscle cells that causes a local or referred pain pattern; may also cause muscle weakness, loss of range of motion, and tingling.

trigger point pressure release:
Sustained pressure, usually with an elbow or self-care tool, on an area identified as having pain-causing dysfunctional muscle tissue. Part of a comprehensive manual therapy protocol.

tui na:
A variety of techniques from traditional Chinese medicine, including massage, joint mobilization, acupressure, moxibustion, and cupping. Evolved from Chinese anmo.

tsubo:
The Japanese name for the deep pressure points along the meridians.

wellness:
The concept of prevention of disease, as opposed to treating the symptom; the wellness philosophy encourages the individual to take charge of his or her own continued health.

yoga:
An ancient healing system using breathing, diet, and stretching postures to promote wellness.

Appendix B: Resources

Organizations

The following is a list of organizations that can help you find a massage therapist, massage school, or massage materials:

Academic Consortium for Complementary and Alternative Health Care (ACCAHC)
www.accahc.org
Alliance for Massage Therapy Education (AFMTE)
www.AFMTE.org
American Massage Therapy Association (AMTA)
www.amtamassage.org
American Organization for Bodywork Therapies of Asia
www.aobta.org
American Reflexology Certification Board (ARCB)
www.arcb.net
Associated Bodywork & Massage Professionals (ABMP)
www.abmp.com
Certification Board for Myofascial Trigger Point Therapists
www.cbmtpt.org
Chicago Center for Myofascial Pain Relief (Advanced Trigger Point Seminars; Education and Training)
www.ChicagoTriggerPointCenter.com
Commission on Massage Therapy Accreditation (COMTA)
www.comta.org
Federation of State Massage Therapy Boards (FSMTB)
www.fsmtb.org
Institute of Complementary Medicine
www.icmedicine.com
International Council of Reflexologists
www.icr-reflexology.org
International Spa Association (ISPA)
www.experienceispa.com
Massage Therapy Foundation (MTF)
www.massagetherapyfoundation.org

National Association of Myofascial Trigger Point Therapists (NAMTPT)

www.namtpt.org

National Certification Board for Therapeutic Massage & Bodywork

www.ncbtmb.com

Society for Oncology Massage

www.s4om.org

Structure for Wounded Warriors (Massage for Veterans)

www.structureforwoundedwarriors.org

Thai Bodywork School of Thai Massage

www.thaibodywork.com

The Trigger Point & Referred Pain Guide

www.triggerpoints.net

Books

Here are a few resources on the subjects covered in this book:

Ackerman, Diane. *A Natural History of the Senses.*

Allen, Tina. *A Modern-Day Guide to Massage for Children.*

Barnett, Libby, and Maggie Chambers. *Reiki Energy Medicine.*

Beck, Mark F. *Milady's Theory and Practice of Therapeutic Massage.*

Biancalana, Mary, et al. *Trigger Point Therapy for Low Back Pain.*

Blate, Michael. *The Natural Healer's Acupressure Handbook.*

Borysenko, Joan. *7 Paths to God.*

Brennan, Barbara Ann. *Hands of Light.*

Cailliet, Rene. *Soft Tissue Pain and Disability.*

Calvert, Robert Noah. *The History of Massage.*

Chaitow, Leon. *Fascial Dysfunction: Manual Therapy Approaches.*

Chaitow, Leon, and Sandy Fritz. *A Massage Therapist's Guide to Lower Back and Pelvic Pain.*

Chopra, Deepak. *Perfect Health.*

Clay, James, and David Pounds. *Basic Clinical Massage Therapy: Integrating Anatomy and Treatment.*

Coulter, David. *Anatomy of Hatha Yoga.*

Davies, Clair. *The Frozen Shoulder Workbook.*

Davies, Clair, and Amber Davies. *The Trigger Point Therapy Workbook, Third Edition.*

Davis, Phyllis R. *The Power of Touch.*

Devereux, Charla, and Bernie Hephrun. *The Perfume Kit.*

Devonshire, Rosalie, and Julie Kelly. *Taking Charge of Fibromyalgia*.

Dougans, Inge. *The Complete Illustrated Guide to Reflexology*.

Eddy, Mary Baker. *Science and Health*.

Ferguson, Lucy Whyte, and Robert Gerwin. *Clinical Mastery in the Treatment of Myofascial Pain*.

Finando, Donna. *Trigger Point Self-Care Manual*.

Franzen, Susanne. *Shiatsu: For Health and Well-Being*.

Fritz, Sandy. *Mosby's Fundamentals of Therapeutic Massage*.

Gach, Michael R., and Carolyn Marco Matzkin. *Acu-Yoga*.

Goodman, Saul. *The Book of Shiatsu*.

Grossman, Gail Boorstein. *Yoga Journal Presents: Restorative Yoga for Life*.

Heath, Alan, and Nicki Bainbridge. *Baby Massage*.

Jackson, Richard. *Holistic Massage*.

Jaffe, Marjorie. *The Muscle Memory Method*.

Jarmey, Chris, and John Tindall. *Acupressure for Common Ailments*.

Judith, Anodea, PhD. *Wheels of Life*.

Kahn, Robert L., and John W. Rowe. *Successful Aging*.

Kirsta, Alix. *The Book of Stress Survival*.

Kushi, Michio, and Edward Esko. *Basic Shiatsu*.

Levine, Barbara. *Your Body Believes Every Word You Say*.

Lidell, Lucy. *The Book of Massage*.

Lidell, Lucy. *The Sensual Body*.

Loewendahl, Evelyn. *The Power of Positive Stretching*.

Loving, Jean E. *Massage Therapy*.

Lu, Henry C. *Chinese Natural Cures*.

Lundberg, Paul. *The Book of Shiatsu*.

Lunny, Vivian, MD. *Aromatherapy*.

Maxwell-Hudson, Clare. *Aromatherapy Massage*.

McCarty, Patrick. *A Beginner's Guide to Shiatsu*.

McClure, Vimala Schneider. *Infant Massage*.

Mitchell, Karyn. *Reiki: A Torch in Daylight*.

Montagu, Ashley. *Touching: The Human Significance of the Skin*.

Mumford, Susan. *The Complete Guide to Massage*.

Muramoto, Naboru. *Healing Ourselves*.

Myss, Caroline. *Anatomy of the Spirit*.

Nelson, Douglas. *The Mystery of Pain*.

O'Keefe, Adele. *The Official Guide to Body Massage*.

Pritchard, Sarah. *Chinese Massage Manual*.

Prudden, Bonnie. *Pain Erasure*.

Rister, Robert. *Japanese Herbal Medicine*.

Roizen, Michael F. *RealAge*.

Rush, Anne Kent. *Romantic Massage*.

Rynerson, Kay. *The Thai Massage Workbook*.

Salvo, Susan G. *Massage Therapy: Principles and Practice*.

Schleip, Robert, et al. *Fascia: The Tensional Network of the Human Body*.

Sharamon, Shalila, and Bodo J. Baginski. *The Chakra Handbook*.

Shaw, Nancy Lee. *Simple Changes to End Chronic Pain*.

Shifflett, Carol. *Migraine Brains and Bodies*.

Starlanyl, Devin. *Fibromyalgia and Chronic Myofascial Pain Syndrome*.

Starlanyl, Devin, and John Sharkey. *Healing Through Trigger Point Therapy*.

Stillerman, Elaine. *Mother Massage*.

Stormer, Chris. *Reflexology: The Definitive Guide*.

Street, Virginia Powell. *Janet Travell, M.D.: White House Physician and Trigger Point Pioneer*.

Tappan, Frances. *Healing Massage Techniques*.

Tortora, Gerard, and Bryan H. Derrickson. *Introduction to the Human Body*.

Travell, Janet, and David Simons. *Travell & Simons' Myofascial Pain and Dysfunction: The Trigger Point Manuals*.

Tucker, Louise. *An Introductory Guide to Reflexology*.

Walters, Lynne. *Kind Touch Massage*.

Werner, Ruth, and Ben E. Benjamin. *A Massage Therapist's Guide to Pathology*.

Westcott, Patsy. *Overcoming Stress*.

Widdowson, Rosalind. *Head Massage*.

Yogananda, Paramahansa. *Autobiography of a Yogi*.

Yu, Winnie, and Michael McNett. *The Everything® Health Guide to Fibromyalgia*.

Zuleger, Julie, and Spring and Faussett. *Happy Muscles Self-Help Guide to Un-knot Your Pain*.

Magazines and Journals

There are a few magazines and journals dedicated to massage:

International Journal of Therapeutic Massage & Bodywork
www.ijtmb.org
Journal of Bodywork and Movement Therapies
www.bodyworkmovementtherapies.com
Massage Australia
www.massageaustralia.com.au

Massage Magazine

www.massagemag.com

Massage Therapy Journal

www.amtamassage.org

Massage Today

www.massagetoday.com

The Pain Practitioner

www.aapainmanage.org

Townsend Newsletter

www.townsendletter.com

Web Sources

The Internet is another good resource for information about massage. Here are a few sites for obtaining equipment, but there are many more:

www.customcraftworks.com (self-care tools, massage tables, and massage chairs)

www.earthlite.com

www.bestmassagetable.com

www.massagenaturals.com

www.massagewarehouse.com

www.motherearthpillows.com (warm flaxseed bags for natural heat and cold)

www.myobuddy.com (massage and trigger point support tool)

www.posturedynamics.com (correction for poor posture and pain)

www.purepro.com (high-quality massage lotion, with or without arnica essential oil)

www.fomentek.com (water bags for soothing muscles)

www.fitball.com (self-care tools, dynamic seating, rehabilitation, massage)

www.pressurepositive.com (self-care tools)

www.triggerpointproducts.com (self-care tools and products for massage therapists)

www.tigertailusa.com (self-care tools)

www.kismetpotions.com (essential oils)

www.sanjevani.net (Ayurveda Healing Clinic and education center)

www.healthandmed.com

Index

31901056936786